Monoclonal Antibodies

Monoclonal Antibodies

KAROL SIKORA

MA, MB, MRCP, FRCR, PhD
Director, Ludwig Institute for Cancer Research;
Honorary Consultant in Radiotherapy and
Oncology, Addenbrooke's and
Hinchingbrooke Hospitals, Cambridge

HOWARD M. SMEDLEY

MB, BS FRCR
Senior Registrar in Radiotherapy and Oncology,
Addenbrooke's Hospital;
former Senior Clinical Scientist,
Ludwig Institute for Cancer Research, Cambridge

With a chapter by

PAUL FINAN
FRCS
Lecturer in Surgery
University of Leeds

and a foreword by

CÉSAR MILSTEIN
FRS

BLACKWELL SCIENTIFIC PUBLICATIONS

OXFORD LONDON EDINBURGH
BOSTON MELBOURNE

© 1984 by
Blackwell Scientific Publications
Editorial offices:
Osney Mead, Oxford, OX2 0EL
8 John Street, London, WC1N 2ES
9 Forrest Road, Edinburgh,
   EH1 2QH
52 Beacon Street, Boston
   Massachusetts 02108, USA
99 Barry Street, Carlton
   Victoria 3053, Australia

First published 1984

Set by Colset Private Limited,
Singapore
Printed and bound in Great Britain
by Butler & Tanner Ltd,
Frome and London

DISTRIBUTORS

USA
   Blackwell Mosby Book
   Distributors, 11830 Westline
   Industrial Drive, St Louis,
   Missouri 63141

Canada
   Blackwell Mosby Book
   Distributors, 120 Melford Drive,
   Scarborough, Ontario, M1B 2X4

Australia
   Blackwell Scientific Book
   Distributors, 31 Advantage Road,
   Highett, Victoria 3190

British Library
Cataloguing in Publication Data

Sikora, Karol
   Monoclonal antibodies.
   1. Antibodies, Monoclonal
   I. Title   II. Smedley, Howard M.
   III. Finan, Paul
   612'.118223   QR186.85

ISBN 0–632–01166–1

TO
SIMON, EMMA, LUCY,
THOMAS AND
ELEANOR

Contents

Foreword

This short book describes the application of monoclonal antibodies in biology and medicine. It outlines the steps necessary to construct monoclonal antibodies and select those suitable for a particular task. Their specificity and constant availability have made them prime reagents in clinical and non-clinical laboratories. The authors have striven hard to explain all the potential areas of application. There are separate chapters on each of the clinical laboratory disciplines where the use of monoclonal antibodies will almost certainly revolutionize many of the current time-consuming assay procedures. Their use as molecular flags in the purification of biologically interesting substances and the analysis of the molecules responsible for differentiation is also described. This in turn leads to a consideration of the problem of cancer — a disease of great interest to biologists and physicians alike.

The book is well illustrated with clear line diagrams. No prior immunological knowledge is necessary to understand the well-written text. The book should be of great benefit to students of all ages who wish to keep abreast with new developments in molecular biology.

César Milstein

Preface

Since their discovery in 1975 monoclonal antibodies have become a key research tool of the biotechnology era, opening up many new fields of biological and clinical research. It is their remarkable specificity that enables them to be used with great precision to identify complex biological molecules. They have led to assays for previously unmeasurable substances; the identification of new cell populations and the uncovering of novel differentiation pathways. Monoclonals are poised to revolutionize all branches of laboratory medicine as well as having exciting therapeutic possibilities for patients with cancer, infectious diseases and auto-immune disorders.

This book provides a background to their development and highlights current areas of progress. As the authors are practising clinicians it is written with a certain bias to clinical medicine. We hope it will be of use to students of medicine and biology as well as physicians who wish to keep abreast of the biotechnology revolution.

We thank our wives Alison and Mary for their editorial assistance; Susan Hamilton and Mary-Ann Starkey for typing and retyping the manuscript; Mark Sinnott for giving us consumer reaction and the artwork; and finally Peter Saugman our publisher for his patience and persistence.

Karol Sikora
Howard Smedley
Cambridge 1983

Chapter 1

What is a Monoclonal Antibody?

In 1975 George Köhler and César Milstein working in the Laboratory of Molecular Biology in Cambridge described a technique to produce endless quantities of antibodies of defined and predictable specificity. This technique has revolutionized the study and practice of immunology as well as providing tools of immense value in many areas of biology and medicine. We will outline later in this book the theoretical and practical considerations in the production of such antibodies along with their application. It must be understood from the outset that monoclonal antibodies (MCA's) do not differ structurally from other antibodies found under natural conditions. The property which makes MCA's unique is that all the molecules in any single preparation are identical. Their reaction with any defined antigen — the opposite partner in the fundamental reaction of immunology — must also be exactly the same each time. It is this constancy in preparation and in effect that makes them so useful. Immunologically complex structures such as cell surfaces may be dissected at a molecular level and studied, piece by piece. The knowledge so gained will have a tremendous impact on our understanding of many diseases and the way in which they are treated.

The immune system

All higher animals have the ability to recognize foreign and potentially harmful molecules entering their bodies. Efforts are made to isolate or expel such foreign molecules. The immune system is the major defence mechanism against substances that have gained entry. A substance capable of exciting such a reaction from the immune system is called an antigen. The body's reaction to the recognition of this antigen is to manufacture a protein called an antibody. An antibody, recognizing an antigen, links to it by a series of chemical bonds. These bonds are individually very weak (non-covalent) but their number overcomes this weakness. The locking of an antibody and its antigen is rather like the linking of two large pieces in a jigsaw puzzle. The combination of the two molecules sets in motion a series of events within the body which

1

Table 1.1. Effects of antibody–antigen interaction

Interaction	Effects
Immune complex formation	Removal of antigen, serum sickness, disease states
Complement activation	Lysis of bacteria or cells
Macrophage activation	Cell lysis
Killer cell activation	Cell lysis
Immunoregulation	Control of immune system

may end in the expulsion of the antigen from the body. These events are listed in Table 1.1.

Antibodies are found in the globulin fraction of the proteins that circulate in the blood and are called immunoglobulins. They are divided into five main classes on the basis of their physical characteristics, such as molecular weight, and are referred to by a letter associated with each class, i.e. IgG, IgA, IgM, IgD and IgE (Table 1.2). Some subclasses have specific physiological functions. IgE is associated with the immune reaction of allergic responses and IgA is the major immunoglobulin component of external body secretions such as lacrimal fluid. IgG is the commonest immunoglobulin found in the circulating plasma and accounts for 75% of the globulin fraction.

As well as producing antibodies, the immune system can also respond through its cellular components. This cellular immunity is largely responsible for the rejection of organ transplants, delayed allergic responses and graft-versus-host reactions. A classical example of cellular immunity is the response to tuberculin, the coat protein of the tubercle bacillus, when injected under the skin. The characteristic red zone of oedema that appears after 48 hr is due to

Table 1.2

Class	Heavy chains	Molecular weight	Relative serum concentration (%)
IgG	γ	150,000	75
IgM	μ	900,000	8
IgA	α	160,000	16
IgD	δ	180,000	< 1
IgE	ϵ	180,000	< 1

local infiltration of activated lymphocytes around the deposited protein. Experiments in mice have shown that the development of cellular immunity is dependent on the presence of the thymus in early life. The thymus is a gland in the upper chest that shrinks after childhood. Lymphocytes conditioned in the thymus are referred to as T-lymphocytes.

Humoral immunity is conferred by the presence of circulating immunoglobulins in tissue fluids. In birds, the lymphocytes that produce circulating antibodies are dependent upon the presence of an organ known as a Bursa of the Fabricius, associated with the large intestine. Although there is no known comparable organ in man, such antibody-producing lymphocytes, which are independent of the thymus, are called B-lymphocytes. MCA production requires that the antibody-producing B-lymphocytes are made immortal in the laboratory, and allowed to continue to synthesize antibodies.

Antibody–antigen interaction

Many molecules are capable of giving rise to an immune response, i.e.

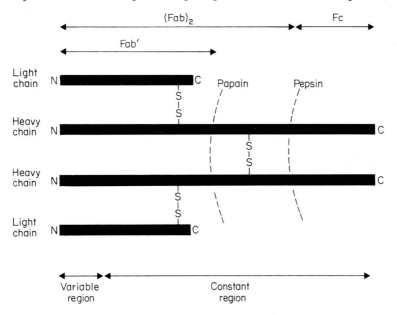

Fig. 1.1. Structure of IgG. The variable region and antigen-binding sites are at the N-terminus of the peptide chains.

3

they are antigens. Each molecule has a unique shape. It is this shape which gives rise to the specificity of an antigen–antibody reaction. Clearly larger and more complex molecules may have several different regions, each of which is capable of accommodating an antibody. Such regions are known as antigenic determinants or epitopes. It is possible for one antigenic molecule to contain several epitopes. Smaller antigens, on the other hand, may possess only one epitope. The basis of the antibody–antigen interaction is the fitting together of two molecules of complementary shape. The shape of the antigen is determined by the three dimensional structure of the molecule. All immunoglobulin molecules have a similar basic structure consisting of two heavy and two light chains held together by disulphide bonds (Fig. 1.1).

Antibodies have areas in the heavy and light chains known as variable regions in which the amino acid sequence of the protein chain varies from one antibody to another. This variation occurs at the N-terminus of the peptide chains. Each different antibody will therefore have a different amino acid sequence and spatial arrangement. It is therefore conceivable that every possible shape presented by an antigen can be accommodated by some antibody produced by the immune system (Fig 1.2). The mechanisms in which such a diverse series of proteins are generated from a limited amount of information encoded in the DNA of an individual has received considerable attention over recent years. The genes that code for different chains of the immunoglobulin are located at different sites of the genome. In addition, there are several constant region and variable region domains within each chain, which are spliced together at a genetic level during lymphocyte differentiation. Each individual has the capacity to manufacture an antibody which will combine with every possible antigen, but the body is only stimulated to manufacture a specific antibody after the introduction of the appropriate antigen. This may occur naturally by ingestion in the gut, by infection with bacteria or virus, or artificially during the process of immunization. Once an antibody has been made, an individual can produce relatively large quantities of it very easily. This is called the 'memory' of the immune system. It was first recognized by the observation that infection with some diseases such as rubella may provide protection against subsequent re-infection.

When an antibody–antigen reaction has occurred several events

4

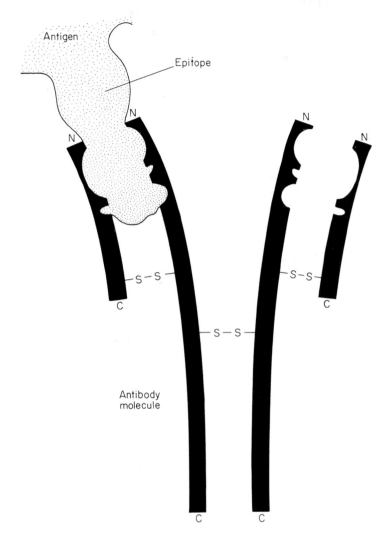

Fig. 1.2. Schematic diagram showing binding of an antigenic determinant to a binding site at the N-terminus of an antibody molecule.

may take place. First, the complex of antibody and antigen may form a molecular lattice which grows in size, and eventually such complexes will be removed from the blood by phagocytic cells. Second, the combination of such molecules can cause the activation of complement, a complex cascade of proteins present in inert form in the blood which, when activated, may cause the lysis of a foreign cell. Alternatively the wandering macrophages of the reticulo-endothelial system may be directed to a specific site in the body and phagocytosis of foreign cells enhanced.

An essential principle of immunology is that each B-lymphocyte may produce only one specific immunoglobulin. This is elegantly outlined in the clonal selection theory. This provides an explanation for features such as immunological memory, the distinction between self and non-self, immunological tolerance, and also auto-immune disease where the body's recognition of self and non-self may break down. The clonal selection theory states that on exposure to an antigen there is a proliferation in the clone of B-lymphocytes responsible for producing the antibody against that antigen. Once proliferation of a clone has occurred, then further exposure to the same antigen results in a rapid and large burst of antibody production accounting for the 'memory' of the immune system. There are certain forbidden clones — those whose secreted antibody would be harmful to the host by interacting with normal human components. By constant immunological stimulation during infancy and childhood, a series of antibody-producing clones of B-cells arise which form the antibody repertoire of an individual. Clearly as every child's antigenic exposure is different in timing and quantity so the repertoire varies between individuals.

Producing a monoclonal antibody

In order to obtain an unlimited supply of a defined antibody to an antigen in the laboratory, all that is required is the isolatation and immortalization of the relevant clone of B-lymphocytes from an animal. The clone could be isolated and grown under laboratory conditions by cell culture. In this way the cloned B-lymphocytes would continue to produce the antibody, which could be collected from the fluid supernatant bathing the cells in culture. However, most attempts to grow clones of B-lymphocytes in the laboratory have failed. What is required therefore is to develop some method by which antibody-producing B-lymphocytes can grow freely and well in laboratory culture.

In the early 1970s it was already possible to grow several types of cell under just such conditions. One type of cell that could be grown easily was a malignancy of B-lymphocytes known as a myeloma or plasmacytoma. These cells have the ability to reproduce themselves indefinitely, unlike their normal non-cancerous counterparts. Furthermore such cells are clonogenic — that is single cells will grow up to form clones either in vitro or when injected into suitable animals. If the property of growth in vitro and clonogenicity from the myeloma cell line could be combined with the property of antibody manufacture from the B-lymphocyte, the possibility of immortalizing defined antibody production could be overcome (Fig. 1.3).

In 1975, Köhler and Milstein demonstrated that myeloma cells could be fused with B-lymphocytes and the resultant hybrids produced antibodies. The technical details and problems of doing this will be explained later. When the fusion process is complete the daughter cells are known as 'hybridomas', i.e. hybrid cells which have inherited some characteristics from both parents and which grow as rapidly malignant cells. The characteristics required, which are actively selected for, are immortality from the malignant myeloma cell and

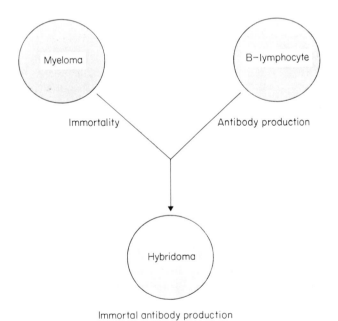

Immortal antibody production

Fig. 1.3. The fusion of a myeloma and an antibody-producing cell results in an immortal antibody-producing hybridoma.

antibody production from the B-lymphocyte. Thus, hybridization techniques allow immunoglobulin-producing cells to be immortalized. However, they do not determine which lymphocyte is being immortalized. To achieve this Köhler and Milstein developed the ingenious technique of immunizing their experimental animal with the antigen of interest. A mouse was immunized by the injection of the antigen — sheep red-blood cells in the first experiment — on several occasions. After several weeks the mouse's immune system would be switching on its own inherent clones of B-lymphocytes which were capable of producing antibodies that recognized the test antigen. The mouse was then killed and lymphocytes collected from the spleen which were used in the fusion process with the myeloma line. In this way it was likely that many of the lymphocytes fused would be secreting the antibody against the antigen of interest. It is important to understand that even using techniques such as this, in which the animal is primed to produce specific antibodies, many lymphocytes will be fused which are producing irrelevant antibodies. When a successful hybridization of myeloma and B-lymphocyte takes place and a colony, or single clone, of hybridoma cells all producing one antibody is established, this antibody is referred to as a monoclonal.

Although the fusion techniques outlined above enable antibodies of defined specificity to be produced in endless quantities, it should be stressed right from the beginning that for every successful antibody which is produced many failed fusions or irrelevant monoclonals will be produced. Many hours of laboratory time are spent to produce a single useful MCA. Some of the reasons for this are obvious. First of all the definition of what is a 'good' monoclonal antibody is arbitrary and depends upon what function is required of it by the investigator. For example, some antibodies may be extremely good at recognizing certain types of lymphocytes in pathological sections and may help the histopathologist in the diagnosis of difficult diseases. However, the staining of such sections may be successful only under certain stringent conditions, such as the use of fresh tissue, and so severely limit the practical application of the antibody to circumstances in which tissue can be collected and examined in a fresh condition. It is therefore important for an investigator to know what he requires of his antibody before deciding which antibodies are good or bad. Further, many antigens against which the investigator is attempting to raise monoclonal antibodies are only weakly immunogenic. The animal's immune system therefore responds poorly to the immunogen and so the incidence of suitable monoclonals is low, thus increasing the workload.

Complex antigens

In biological situations, single epitope molecules are rarely encountered. Much more common is a complex structure, such as a foreign cell, which contains on its surface many hundreds or even thousands of antigenic determinants. Furthermore, not all of these determinants are expressed at all times on the cell surface. It is well known that many antigens are only expressed during phases of rapid cell division or under certain physical conditions. In cancer cells it is common for antigens to be expressed which are normally only encountered during fetal development (the oncofetal antigens). Therefore if such a complex mixture of molecules is injected into an animal, each of the antigenic determinants causes the host animal to produce a specific antibody and the serum of such an animal, if examined at a later date, will contain many different types of antibody, i.e. a polyclonal antiserum. Although such sera have been examined in the past for evidence of immune response to malignancy and infection, it is clear that the very complexity of the antigen means that discovering differences, for example, between normal cells and their malignant counterparts is extremely difficult, if not impossible. There is considerable evidence from experimental work that malignant cells are capable of exciting a definite, but weak, immune response from their host and this implies that at least some antigenic determinants differ from those on the normal cell. However, if we use the monoclonal antibody technology to produce antibodies against the same complex cell surface, we can examine each antibody in turn. In this way it has been found that the great majority of determinants are shared by normal and malignant cells. However, it is possible that an antibody may be discovered which is capable of recognizing an antigen present on a malignant cell, which is not present on its normal counterpart. Subtle differences between normal and malignant cells may be identified and exploited for diagnostic and therapeutic use. However, practice has shown that although such differences may exist, and indeed be recognized, the antigens discovered may also exist on other body tissues, e.g. antibodies raised against human colorectal cancer may recognize white cells in the bone marrow as well as the malignant tumour. A similar approach can also be used in distinguishing different types of micro-organisms which cause infectious disease. The rapid and precise diagnosis of both bacterial and virus disease is thus possible.

Specificity

It has already been stated that spatial arrangement or molecular conformation determines the recognition of antigen by antibody. If, however, the shape which is recognized is very small — part of a structure rather than a whole structure — then the chances increase that a similar shape may be found in another molecule. It is obvious that if the shape to be recognized by the antibody is sufficiently small, the likelihood of this confusion occurring must be greatly increased. An antibody which is too specific may thus have little use in that the particular shape recognized may already be widely distributed on different molecules. There clearly must be an optimal specificity determined by the size and configuration of the binding site.

Antibody characteristics

The strength with which an antibody binds to an antigen is known as its affinity. Depending on the practical use which is required of the antibody, it is possible that strong binding of antibody to an antigen may be, under different circumstances, a good or a bad thing. Under normal conditions the antibody–antigen interaction occurs so that the body may eliminate potentially harmful substances. Secondary reactions take place so that the complexed antigen may be recognized and eliminated. However, as will be seen later, in clinical practice it may be desirable to introduce an antibody into a patient in order to find a particular type of cell or tissue. Under these circumstances clearly it would be very undesirable if the binding characteristics of the monoclonal antibody to the normal tissue were such that complement fixation occurred and the antibody caused the death of a normal tissue. In other circumstances, monoclonal antibodies may be introduced into patients in order to eliminate drugs or poisons. Here it is clearly essential that they should retain the ability to help in the excretion of the unwanted antigens.

Choice of animal for antibody production

Antibodies are prepared by immunizing an animal so that its own immune system is triggered to produce antibodies against the antigens of interest. In the laboratory, mice and rats have been studied extensively. The animal is immunized at weekly intervals for 3 or 4 weeks with the antigen to be studied, and is finally killed and lymphocytes taken. In practice, this is done by removing the spleen of the animal, which is a rich source of lymphocytes, and preparing a fresh single-cell suspension from which lymphocytes can subsequently be isolated. Similarly the myeloma lines used are also of mouse and rat origin and established in tissue culture. An early observation was that inter-species hybridization is unreliable as resulting daughter cells tend to be unstable in their genetic constitution. Therefore mouse lymphocytes are fused with mouse myeloma lines and rat lymphocytes with rat myeloma lines.

In this book we are principally concerned with the application of the monoclonal antibody technology to medical practice. For this it would be desirable to have human monoclonal antibodies, i.e. MCA's prepared by the fusion of human B-lymphocytes with a human myeloma line. Until recently this has not proved possible. Firstly, it is clearly not always ethically possible to immunize human subjects with antigens of interest such as toxins, bacteria or malignant cells. Secondly, there have been great difficulties in producing stable, infection-free cell lines of human myelomas in culture. However, recent advances have made the production of stable human myeloma lines feasible whilst immunization problems have been overcome by obtaining for fusion lymphocytes from the lymph nodes of patients known to be suffering from particular diseases, removed routinely at operation. These cells are fused with a human myeloma line and stable human hybrid cells obtained. When subsequent re-administration of these MCA's is contemplated for diagnostic or therapeutic purposes, human antibodies would have the overwhelming advantage that as a naturally occurring human protein they would be unable to excite an immunological reaction in the recipient, which is always a worry when administering rat or mouse proteins.

Conclusion

Monoclonal antibodies are immunoglobulins which are of immense value and interest because the method of their production allows the manufacture of endless quantities of a single antibody against an antigen which may be specially selected. Not only does this open the door for many advances to be made in our understanding of the basic principles of the working of the immune system, but also offers the exciting possibility that such knowledge will enable new methods of diagnosis and therapy to be pioneered in the next few years.

Further reading

Hobart M.J. & McConnell I. (1982) *The Immune System.* Blackwell Scientific Publications, Oxford.

Kohler G. & Milstein C. (1975) Continuous cultures of fused cells producing antibodies of predefined specificity. *Nature,* **256,** 495–497.

Lachmann P.J. & Peters D.K. (1982) *Clinical Aspects of Immunology.* Blackwell Scientific Publications, Oxford.

McMichael A.J. & Fabre J.W. (1982) *Monoclonal Antibodies in Clinical Medicine.* Academic Press, London.

Mitchell M.S. & Oettgen H.F. (1982) *Hybridomas in Cancer Diagnosis and Therapy.* Raven Press, New York.

Chapter 2

Making a Monoclonal Antibody

The antigen

Monoclonal antibodies can be made to any substance that will be recognized as an antigen by the cells in the immune system of an animal. As explained in Chapter 1, when a single substance or a mixture of substances is injected into an animal, a series of antibodies are made which recognize certain components in the antigen. These components are called antigenic determinants or epitopes. The polyclonal antibodies produced are a complex series of immunoglobulins which recognize a whole range of different epitopes. The first step in producing a monoclonal antibody to a defined antigen is to make a suitable preparation of the antigen for immunization. In some cases it will be possible to make a completely pure preparation using a chemical technique. An example would be the development of a monoclonal antibody for assaying a drug such as digoxin. This is a drug which is used commonly to treat patients with heart disease. Purified digoxin can be used to immunize animals so that anti-digoxin antibodies are produced. In many instances, however, a pure substance cannot be used, but a mixture of either partially purified or even very impure substances are all that is available. This was the case in the preparation of monoclonal antibodies to interferon after its partial purification. A mixture of substances which contained interferon was used to immunize animals and the correct monoclonal antibodies selected by analysis after cloning. In some cases the position is even more complex. In trying to make monoclonal antibodies to molecules that are uniquely present on cancer cell surfaces, whole tumour cells or cell surface preparations of such cells are used as immunogens. These contain a range of molecules which are also present on normal cells. The aim of making monoclonal antibodies is to produce a reagent which can distinguish those molecules that are present uniquely on the cancer cell, and not on normal cells, and to use such antibodies to help in the treatment of cancer patients.

Immunization

Animals are immunized by injecting the antigen either subcutaneously or into the peritoneal cavity surrounding the intestine. At the same time the immune system of the animal may be stimulated by injecting a mixture of powerful immune stimulants. The most commonly used is Freund's adjuvant. This mixture of dead tuberculosis organisms in a fatty base has the effect of priming the immune system to recognize avidly any antigen injected with the mixture. Animals are normally injected on several occasions, usually at weekly intervals, to ensure good immune stimulation. With each successive immunization there is increased stimulation of the B-lymphocyte clones within the animal responding to the antigen. The final boost of antigen is given intra-venously usually 3 days prior to the collection of spleen cells to ensure that the B-cell clones of interest are maximally stimulated. The cells that grow best after fusion are those that are rapidly dividing. It has been shown that the time of maximal growth rate of immune stimu-lated cells is 3 days after immunization. The reason for the intra-venous injection is to give a high peak dose of antigen. In this way a large cohort of cells are stimulated simultaneously.

Fusion

After killing the animal, its abdomen is opened up and the spleen removed and placed in tissue culture fluid. From now on everything must be done under sterile conditions to prevent bacteria and fungi getting into the tissue culture dishes in the laboratory and causing widespread infection. To prevent this the fluid in which cells are now kept contains antibiotics, usually penicillin and streptomycin, to prevent bacterial growth. The spleens are teased apart, releasing the lymphocytes within them. Clumps of membrane are removed by allow-ing the suspension of spleen cells and debris from the surface of the spleen to settle, leaving a preparation of single cells in tissue culture fluid.

The spleen contains not only lymphocytes but also an abundance of red cells. These can be removed by centrifugation on a dense fluid — Ficoll. Ficoll is placed in a centrifuge tube and the spleen cells gently layered on top using a Pasteur pipette. The tube is now centrifuged for 20 min at a low speed, usually 400 g. The red cell clump sinks to the

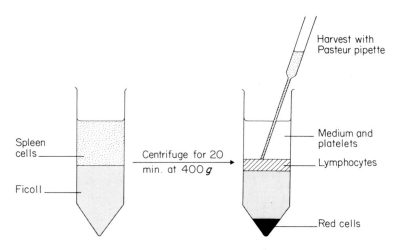

Fig. 2.1. The use of Ficoll to separate viable lymphocytes from a spleen cell suspension containing red cells and platelets.

bottom, together with any dead cells. The lymphocytes remain at the top of the Ficoll, forming a pale white band (Fig. 2.1). The fluid in which the spleen cells were suspended collects above the lymphocytes. The lymphocytes can be harvested using a Pasteur pipette and washed by centrifugation. These cells are now mixed with a myeloma, which is freshly prepared, ready for fusion. Like all malignant cells, myeloma cells have the capacity for infinite replication. There are several different types of myeloma line available for fusion obtained from mice, rats or humans. One vital feature of such myeloma lines is an in-built destruction mechanism so that myeloma cells that have not fused can be destroyed easily after the fusion process. Approximately equal numbers of myeloma cells and spleen lymphocytes, from the immunized animal, are mixed together in the presence of polyethylene glycol. Originally a virus was used at this stage called Sendai virus but this is troublesome to keep in the laboratory and its use has been almost totally replaced by polyethylene glycol (PEG). PEG is similar to substances used in antifreeze solution to prevent freezing in car radiators. It destroys the surface tension forces which normally cause cells to repel each other when mixed in a test tube. In the presence of PEG, cells can mix intimately. Their membranes fuse allowing the nucleus of one cell to enter the cytoplasm of its neighbour.

A variety of tricks are employed in order to increase the frequency of the fusion process. One is to put another substance called dimethylsulphoxide (DMSO) in the fusion mixture along with PEG. This also increases the closeness of the contact between cells during fusion and increases the chances of success. Both DMSO and PEG are very poisonous to cells and so the timing of the cells' exposure to these substances is critical. Normally cells are kept in the mixture of these chemicals for only a few minutes. During this time the closeness of the cells is increased by pelleting gently by centrifugation for 5 min. The chemicals are diluted by fresh tissue culture fluid and the cells washed. After the fusion the cells are plated out into tissue culture dishes. The mixture now consists of unfused myeloma cells, unfused lymphocytes and hybridomas — the hybrid lymphocyte-myeloma cells.

Selection

Of course not all the myeloma cells will have fused. Indeed, the majority will remain growing healthily in an unfused state. As these cells grow faster than the hybridomas they would rapidly outgrow them. Therefore a self-destruct mechanism is operated. This entails changing the composition of the tissue culture medium as explained in Fig. 2.2. The myeloma cells used for fusion are specially selected by growing them in the presence of a drug called 8-azaguanine. There are several variants of this technique but the principles are identical. The myeloma cells are normally killed by azaguanine but some become resistant to the effects of this drug by switching off permanently the

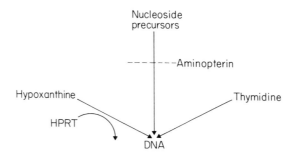

Fig. 2.2. Principles of the HAT selection to destroy unfused myeloma cells after hybridization.

production of an enzyme called hypoxanthine phosphoribosyl transferase (HPRT). Cells are said to be HPRT negative after this selection.
When such HPRT negative cells are grown in a mixture of
hypoxanthine, aminopterin and thymidine (HAT medium) the cells will
die because they can no longer synthesize DNA. The aminopterin
blocks the main pathway for purine and pyrimidine synthesis — the
building blocks of DNA. Normal cells which possess HPRT can utilize
the hypoxanthine to make purines, and the thymidine to make pyri-
midines. HPRT-negative cells cannot do this and so die as the enzyme
HPRT is instrumental in this process.

If we now consider the cells growing out of the fusion mixture; the
normal lymphocytes from the immunized animal's spleen cannot grow
in tissue culture for more than a few days and will therefore die out
naturally. The parent myeloma lacking HPRT will not grow in the HAT
selection medium. However, hybridoma cells will possess the ability to
grow from the myeloma cells, and the HPRT genes from the lymphocytes with which they have fused. Thus the hybridomas will grow
successfully even in the HAT selection medium.

Cloning

If all the hybridoma cells that occurred after a fusion were grown up
together, then a mixture of antibodies would be released similar to
those found in the serum of the whole animal. The trick in producing
monoclonal antibodies comes in isolating single cells and allowing
these to grow up as a clone — each cell being an exact replica of
others. In this way only one immunoglobulin molecule will be secreted.
However, there is one snag; cells do not like to grow in isolation. The
biggest stress in the whole process of making monoclonal antibodies is
in getting single cells to clone, in other words to become many cells by
replication. Once a cell has divided a few times it becomes easy for it
to continue its growth. It is getting the first few cells which is the major
problem. A variety of techniques are used to overcome this. The first is
to add 'feeder' cells, which in a sense make the single cell about to
divide feel at home with other cells which have already grown up. A
second method is to put cells into a very rich tissue culture fluid right
from the start.

Both methods probably work by providing a range of small
molecules known as growth factors that are required for cells to

17

divide. We know little about their structure but they are clearly important in allowing cells to clone. There are two strategies used for
cloning cells in practice (Fig. 2.3). One is the technique of limiting dilution. The suspension of hybrids is diluted and distributed into a series
of sterile wells, usually in plastic dishes. The dilution is calculated so
that the volume of fluid being placed in each well will contain on
average a single cell. Of course some wells will receive no cells and no
growth will occur, and some more than one cell — so that oligoclonal
antibodies will result. After growing up, the initial cloning process can
be repeated several times to ensure true monoclonality.

The second method of cloning is by growth in a solid medium such

Limiting dilution

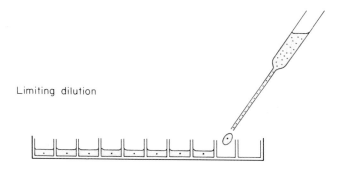

Cloning in gel

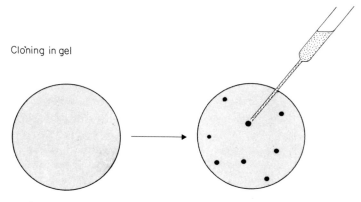

Fig. 2.3. Cloning techniques to obtain cloned hybridomas.

as agarose gel. A variety of gels exist which after the addition of appropriate factors such as serum, amino acids, and antibiotics will support the growth of cells. Cells divide to form clusters that look like tiny spheres. As the medium is semi-solid these spheres can be picked by a fine Pasteur pipette. The cluster can be gently broken by swishing it up and down in the pipette and plated out into a microwell for further culture. Many clones can be isolated in this way and grown up for subsequent analysis.

Screening for antibody

In the process of fusion, the whole spleen of the animal has been used as a source of lymphocytes. Despite the stimulation of the immune system by prior immunization with the antigen of interest, many of the lymphocytes that fuse will be producing antibodies directed against antigens not of interest. Even with the best immunization schedules against a potent antigen, less than 5% of the splenocytes will be producing specific antibodies. To select the relevant hybrids the laborious process of screening each supernatant for antibody activity is required. This is first performed prior to cloning to ensure that only wells containing antibody-secreting hybrids are used. There are many assays available to detect antibodies. An essential feature of the screening assay is that it must be simple and cheap, as it is likely to be performed on many occasions during the production of a monoclonal antibody. A variety of such assays are available.

Binding assays

The simplest assays depend on the ability of a monoclonal antibody to bind to its antigen. The complex is washed to remove any non-specifically bound antibody. The binding reaction can then be detected by using a second antibody which reacts with the first. In the case of a mouse hybridoma system, using a mouse myeloma fused with immunized mice splenocytes, the detector antibody would be rabbit anti-mouse immunoglobulin (produced by immunizing rabbits with immunoglobulin extracted from mouse serum). The second antibody is tagged with either a radioactive isotope that can be detected by a radioactivity counter or an enzyme that will cause a colour change after the addition of appropriate substrates. The production of anti-tetanus toxin antibodies will be used as an example (Fig. 2.4).

Purified tetanus toxin is used to immunize mice prior to fusion. The hybrids are grown up and an assay for mouse anti-tetanus antibody developed. Purified toxin can be immobilized by adsorption to a plastic dish containing many small wells. The process of adsorption is quite non-specific, but extremely useful in developing assays for soluble antigens. A dilute solution (around 10 μg/ml) of antigen is added to each well and left for 3 hr. This process is often carried out at 4°C as this increases the rate of adsorption whilst preserving the integrity of complex antigens. After this time any non-adsorbed antigen is removed by simply turning the microwell plate upside down and flicking out any fluid. The wells are filled with buffered saline and the flicking process repeated. After several such washes saline containing a protein such as bovine serum albumin is added and allowed to bathe the wells for 1 hr. The protein saturates any adsorption sites on the plastic, so preventing non-specific sticking later in the assay. The remainder of the assay is also performed in a medium containing a protein to prevent this non-specific effect. Plates with antigens bound can be prepared in large quantities and stored frozen, ready for use when hybridomas appear.

A small amount of hybridoma supernatant is added to a well. As there are ninety-six wells on each plate then clearly ninety-six supernatants can be screened in one assay. If anti-tetanus toxin antibody is present it will stick to the·antigen on the plate. After 1 hr at 4°C the plate is washed with saline by inverting and flicking, and radio-

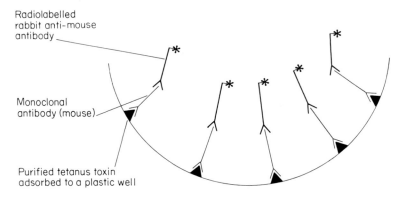

Radiolabelled
rabbit anti-mouse
antibody

Monoclonal
antibody (mouse)

Purified tetanus toxin
adsorbed to a plastic well

Fig. 2.4. Radioimmunoassay for screening for anti-tetanus toxin MCA's.

labelled rabbit anti-mouse immunoglobulin added. [125]Iodine is the usual isotope used in this radioimmunoassay. After a further 1 hr at 4°C, and a further wash to remove unstuck antibody the wells are dried by heating. The plastic wells can be cut with an electrically heated wire which melts the plastic in its path. The wells are placed in small tubes and the radioactivity present in each well determined using a gamma counter. Where antibody has bound to the tetanus toxin there will be increased radioactivity. Of course negative controls (no added antibody) and positive controls (diluted whole serum from the immunized mouse) must be used to ensure the validity of the assay. A further modification used in screening large numbers of supernatants is to put a covered piece of photographic film in direct apposition to the back of the dried microwell plate. Where the ^{125}I has bound in high concentration a dark spot will appear on the developed film. In this way the position of the wells containing antibody can be recorded and the hybridomas selected for cloning and expansion.

Recently many laboratories have used enzyme-linked immuno-absorbent assays (ELISA) in the primary and secondary screening processes. These assays have the advantage of not using any radioactivity, with its associated dangers to health. Instead of tagging the detector antibody (rabbit anti-mouse immunoglobulin) with ^{125}I, an enzyme such as alkaline phosphatase is used. By adding appropriate substrates a colour change will occur which is often clearly visible to the naked eye. Precise measurement can be made by using a spectrophotometer — the so-called ELISA reader machines. In this way the quantity of immunoglobulin in hybridoma supernatants which binds to the antigen of interest can be determined.

Immunohistology

Although radioimmunoassay and ELISA form the basis of most laboratory screening programmes, other possibilities exist. Much will depend on what the desired antibody is to be used for. If, for example, a search is being made for an antibody useful to a pathologist in identifying a certan tissue in biopsy samples from patients, then the primary screening process may involve an immunohistology reaction (cf. Chapter 4). In this way, not only will the screening process select those antibodies which recognize the antigen concerned, but also their ability to perform under the conditions of interest. It is because of the monoclonality of these antibodies that problems can arise in their practical application. In a polyclonal antisera, at least a proportion of the individual immunoglobulin molecules with antigen-binding capacity will have the correct secondary properties which are useful in immunohistology. This may not be the case when a single homogenous set of immunoglobulin molecules is used.

Cytotoxicity

If the purpose of a monoclonal antibody is to kill cells then clearly a cytotoxic screening assay is essential. Antibodies can kill cells in two ways; by activating a cascade of factors in serum called complement; or by attracting to its binding site a population of lymphocytes called killer or K-cells. In both cases the antibody provides the specificity.of recognition whilst the complement or K-cells provide the killing mechanism — simply by punching holes in the targets' cell surface. Cytotoxic activity of an antibody is usually determined by radioactive chromium release assays (Fig. 2.5). Target cells are grown in tissue culture and incubated in sodium chromate made from radioactive chromium (^{51}Cr). The cells can now be regarded as bags of radioactivity which if punctured will release measurable amounts of ^{51}Cr. Antibody is added for 1 hr and the cells washed by centrifugation. Serum containing complement or a population of lymphocytes containing K-cells is added. If antibody has bound then chromium will be released into the fluid bathing the cells. After a further hour the damaged cells are pelleted and the amount of radioactivity released

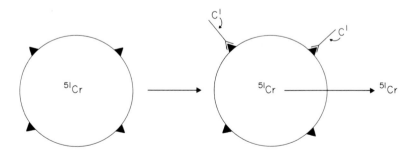

Fig. 2.5. Assay of cell killing by release of radioactive chromium (^{51}Cr) from cells in presence of antibody and complement (C^1).

into the supernatant determined on a gamma counter. An index called specific cytotoxicity can be calculated, by determining the ratio between the counts released during the assay and the counts released maximally by the addition of detergent from which the background control has been subtracted.

Immunochemistry

A further screening method which is being used increasingly is the precipitation of antibody in test supernatants with soluble antigen and the subsequent precipitation of the resultant complex. If the antigen is labelled with a radioactive marker, information about the size distribution of the antigen recognized by a particular antibody can be obtained at the same time. Further refinements are the blotting techniques developed to detect hybridization between complementary sequences of nucleotides on DNA or RNA. Originally described by Dr E. Southern in Edinburgh, the solid phase hybridization of one complementary sequence of DNA to another was called Southern blotting. When used for hybridizing RNA to DNA the name Northern blotting is used (although this technique was described by an investigator called Alwine). To continue this little joke amongst molecular biologists, the solid phase hybridization of two proteins, based on the non-covalent binding occurring by the specific interaction of antibody and its antigen, is universally called Western blotting (Fig. 2.6). This form of screening is particularly useful for detecting antibodies against a complex mixture of molecules such as those found on a cell surface.

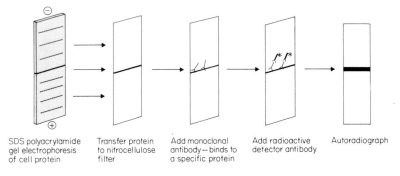

| SDS polyacrylamide gel electrophoresis of cell protein | Transfer protein to nitrocellulose filter | Add monoclonal antibody—binds to a specific protein | Add radioactive detector antibody | Autoradiograph |

Fig. 2.6. The technique of Western blotting for screening for MCA activity.

Let us take the example of carcino-embryonic antigen (CEA); a large 180,000 daltons glycoprotein found on the surface of some colorectal cancer cell lines. Monoclonal antibodies can be raised by immunizing animals with the injection of tumour cells and producing hybridomas. Membranes from the immunizing cell line can be purified, solubilized in detergent, and electrophoresed on an agarose gel. In this way the large molecules will migrate only slowly and end up near the starting line whilst small molecules will flow more rapidly down the gel. Bands of the different proteins in the cell surface will therefore come to lie in positions which reflect their size and shape. A sample of each protein on the gel can be transferred to a nitrocellulose filter or blot. Blotting can be done many times, so that many test pieces of nitrocellulose filter with exactly the same proteins bound can be made. Antibody supernatants are now added, incubated for 1 hr, and washed off. The binding of antibody to its antigen is detected by adding a radiolabelled second antibody exactly as described for radioimmunoassay. The binding of this second antibody is recognized by laying a piece of photographic film against the dried blot and developing it (autoradiography). Not only can the binding of antibody be detected by this technique but also the molecular size of the recognized antigen determined. If monoclonal antibodies to CEA are required then clearly those binding in the 180,000 molecular weight region on the blotted filter must be searched for.

Monoclonal antibody production

By painstakingly screening, cloning and rescreening, hybridomas will be obtained which produce the antibody of interest. There are many pitfalls for the unwary on the way. Tissue culture is notoriously prone to infection by bacteria, fungi, yeasts and also the ubiquitous intracellular pathogen, the mycoplasma. The quality of the fetal calf serum used to support the cells varies between different batches, even if obtained from the same supplier. Myeloma stocks that are growing rapidly and well can suddenly stop growing — a most perplexing and irritating experience for a hybridoma laboratory. Some batches of polyethylene glycol inexplicably refuse to produce hybrids. Even after successful hybridization problems can arise. Most workers rapidly freeze down, in liquid nitrogen, any hybrids producing interesting antibodies for fear of subsequent loss. Cells can be stored indefinitely by freezing at $-196\,^{\circ}$C in liquid nitrogen. Before freezing, cells which are in good health are washed and placed in medium containing either glycerol or dimethyl sulphoxide. These substances prevent the formation of ice crystals in the cells, with resultant damage to intra-cellular organelles. The cells are frozen slowly usually by dropping the temperature at a rate of $1\,^{\circ}$C/min until $-20\,^{\circ}$C is reached.

Once the correct hybridoma line has been obtained an unlimited supply of supernatant containing antibody can be collected. In order to obtain a high concentration of antibody, hybridomas are grown as ascites; that is, as a suspension of tumour cells within the peritoneal cavity of a mouse or rat. Very high titres of antibody can be produced in this way. It is of course important to use the same strain of animal as that of both the parent myeloma and immunized lymphocyte donor so that rejection across histocompatibility barriers, e.g. H-2 in mice, does not occur. To increase the ability of hybridomas to grow in the peritoneal cavity, pristane, an irritant organic solvent is used to prime the mice. This is given intraperitoneally several weeks prior to injection of the cells. This damages the lining of the peritoneum making it a better environment for the hybridoma cells to grow. Ascitic fluid can be collected, centrifuged to remove cells, and aliquoted for future use.

If highly purified monoclonal antibody is required, e.g. for injection into patients, then the growth of cells in large volumes of medium can be performed in roller cultures. The use of media which contain no serum simplifies the purification process. The immunoglobulin is precipitated from spent tissue culture fluid with ammonium sulphate — at a concentration of 50% w/v. The precipitate is redissolved in buffered saline and purified by either affinity columns using immo-bilized protein-A or anti-mouse antibody, or by ion-exchange chromatography. The latter technique has the advantage of being applicable to any antibody without the need for further special reagents. The dissolved ammonium sulphate precipitate is loaded onto a column of diethyl amino-ethyl cellulose (DEAE) in the absence of any salt. The ionic strength of the eluting buffer is gradually increased by a salt gradient apparatus. As the concentration of salt increases, pro-teins with different ionic charges are sequentially eluted. In this way the antibody of interest can be separated from other proteins in the tissue culture supernatant. Purified antibodies or their relatively impure supernatants can be stored indefinitely by freezing. Furthermore many monoclonal antibodies will remain functional for long periods of time even at room temperature. This facilitates their inter-laboratory transfer.

Conclusion

The individual steps in monoclonal antibody production are simple but their integration into a working monoclonal factory is incredibly time-

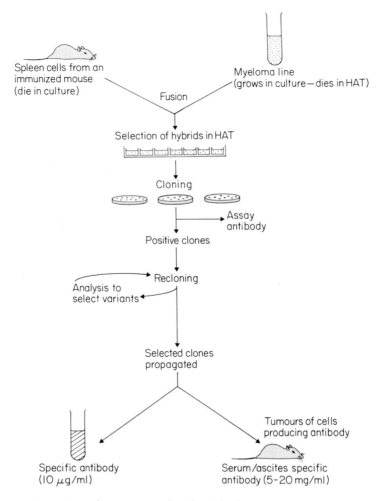

Fig. 2.7. Steps in making a monoclonal antibody.

consuming (Fig. 2.7). The most laborious part of the process is the screening, and automated devices for this are now beginning to appear. It is quite likely that a monoclonal antibody against every possible epitope has already been made, with the hybridoma cells lying dormant in laboratory freezers around the world. Workers that have tried to make monoclonal antibodies to one antigen have ended up with useful reagents against other proteins. A good example is the manufacture and selection of antibodies to human colorectal cancer cells which yielded a set of good blood group typing reagents. To overcome this, laborious search techniques are now being developed to select those B-lymphocytes producing the antibody of interest prior to fusion.

Further reading

Bastin J., Kirkley J. & McMichael A.J. (1982) Production of Monoclonal Antibodies: A practical guide. In: *Monoclonal Antibodies in Clinical Medicine* (Eds A.J. McMichael & J.W. Fabre), p. 503. Academic Press, London.

Kennett R.H. (1982) Cloning of Hybridomas. In: *Monoclonal Antibodies*. (Eds R.H. Kennett, T.J. McKearn & K.B. Bechtol) Plenum Press, New York.

Littlefield J.W. (1964) Selection of hybrids from matings of fibroblasts *in vitro* and their presumed recombinants. *Science*, **145**, 709.

Milstein C. Adetugbo K., Cowan N.J., Kohler G., Secher D. & Wilde C.D. (1976) Somatic cell genetics of antibody producing cells. *Cold Spring Harbor Symp. Quant. Biol.* **41**, 793.

Reading C.L. (1982) Theory and methods for immunization in culture and monoclonal antibody production. *J. Immunol.* **53**, 261–271.

Sharon J., Morrison S.L. & Kabat E.A. (1979) Detection of specific hybridoma clones by replica immunoadsorption of their secreted antibodies. *Proc. Natl. Acad. Sci.* **46**, 1420.

Chapter 3

Biochemistry

Biochemistry aims to understand the chemical contents of living cells and their inter-relationships. Conventionally molecular biology is the term applied to the study of large molecules and their interaction, whereas biochemistry is confined to the smaller molecules. Besides telling us more about how cells work, biochemistry has become as essential tool in modern medicine. A variety of disease states produce abnormalities in body fluids such as blood, urine and cerebrospinal fluid, that can be easily measured in the clinical biochemistry laboratory. Such assays are vital in the management of patients with a wide variety of diseases. To the scientist trying to understand how cells work, and to the physician devising new methods to assess disease states in patients, precise assays for biological molecules are vital. Assays for individual biochemical compounds are also essential for their identification and further purification. Once an effective assay is produced for a particular compound, it can be purified using conventional biochemical techniques such as ultracentrifugation, exclusion chromatography, and ion-exchange chromatography. Furthermore, if specific reagents can be made that will bind biochemical compounds, then by fixing these reagents to a solid matrix, a rapid single step purification method can be devised. This is the basis of affinity chromatography.

Assays

Assays form the cornerstone of the work of the biochemistry laboratory. A variety of techniques are available to measure molecules. Some are based on physical properties, for example the ability of a molecule to migrate to a certain position on a gel because of its size and charge (electrophoresis). Other assays depend on the way in which a compound equilibrates within a chromatography column. Many smaller molecules can be assayed accurately using high pressure liquid chromatography, in which mixtures of molecules are analysed by their position as they elute from separation on an inert matrix under pressure. Unfortunately, many biologically interesting molecules have very similar physical properties and are present in only minute quantities within cells and clinical samples.

Biological activity can be used to assess the number of such molecules present. Interferon, for example, can be measured by its ability to inhibit viral replication. Tissue culture fibroblasts are plated out on plastic dishes and vesicular stomatitis virus added. In the absence of interferon, cytopathic effects will be seen with patches of dying cells appearing within the monolayer of tissue-cultured cells. The addition of increasing quantities of interferon, prior to adding the virus to the system, reduces this cytopathic effect. Such biological assays for interferon have been in use since its discovery 25 years ago. A variety of hormones and pharmacologically active substances can be measured by bioassay. Drugs that affect muscle function can be assayed by the contraction of isolated frog muscle. An example of a clinically used bioassay is that for antibiotics. Many modern antibiotics have toxic effects on kidney and liver. It is therefore important in patients who have impaired kidney and liver function to asess the amount of antibiotic present in the serum. To do this, serum is collected from a patient after the administration of the drug, and plated out on bacteria that have a defined sensitivity to the antibiotic being tested. The amount present is proportional to the number of bacteria being destroyed during the experiment. Unfortunately, bioassays have many problems, they require a source of biological material, frog muscle, bacteria, vesicular stomatitis virus, all of which show variations on different occasions. If reliable results are to be obtained the assays require standardization, individually, each time they are used. They are therefore costly to perform and require considerable skill in maintaining their quality control.

A second method of assaying biologically interesting molecules is to measure their function. Enzymes and coenzymes are readily measured in this way. To measure the amount of alkaline phosphatase in the serum of a patient, serum is taken, and a phosphate containing substrate added. On exposure to the enzyme, the substrate is hydrolysed releasing a coloured product. Unfortunately, many biologically interesting molecules do not have such easily measured functions.

Antisera that specifically recognize individual molecules have been of great use in assay of these molecules. Such antisera are produced by conventional immunization of animals and then used in a variety of immunoassay procedures. The basic principle in all immunoassays is that the antibody binds specifically to its anitgen. A substance can be measured either by competition with a radiolabelled antigen or by determining the amount of immune complex formed by the combination of antibody with the substance. The problems inherent in conventional immunoassays are those of polyclonal antibodies. As outlined in Chapter 1 these include the problems of specificity and batch-to-batch variation of different antisera. Highly immunized animals, such as rabbits, guinea-pigs and sheep, are often used as a source of antisera. However, these animals eventually die. Several regularly performed clinical assays, using conventional antisera, require complete re-standardization when the animal producing the antisera dies. Monoclonal antibodies obviate this problem. Unlimited quantities of a standard antibody can be obtained.

The problem of affinity

The binding of an antigen to an antibody is mediated by non-covalent bonding (hydrogen bonds; van der Waals bonds; hydrophobic bonds; and electrostatic interactions). Such forces are individually very weak but fairly strong in total, and the binding is reversible. The affinity of an antibody reflects the degree of complementarity of an antibody to a single antigen binding site. It is independent of the number of binding sites present on a molecule for an antibody. The reversible binding reaction between an antibody and a single antigenic determinant can be expressed as

$$Ag + Ab \rightleftharpoons AgAb.$$

The equilibrium reached depends on the relative concentrations of the antibody and antigen and the strength of their interaction. This strength can be determined mathematically as an affinity constant (K).

$$K = \frac{[Ag.Ab] \times [Ab]}{[Ag]}$$

This affinity constant K can easily be measured. There is another factor involved in how well an antibody binds to its target antigen. This is the avidity of an antibody. Most antibodies have multiple antigenic sites (epitopes) for binding. If an antibody also has more than one antigen binding site (in the case of IgG two and in the case of IgM five) then these molecules will be more likely to lock tightly onto their target antigen. If the affinity of the binding sites in IgG are the same as those in an IgM molecule recognizing the same determinants on a polymeric protein, then the IgM will bind more tightly, despite its identical affinity constant (Fig. 3.1). Polyclonal antisera contain a variety of antibodies that react to the epitopes expressed on the antigen used as an immunogen. Clearly some of these antibodies will

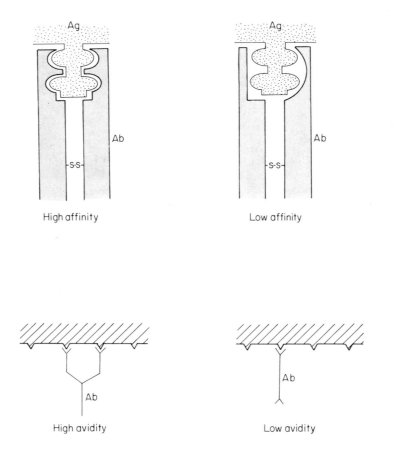

Fig. 3.1. The affinity of an antibody depends upon its closeness of fit with its antigen whilst the avidity is dependent upon the number of binding sites with which it can make contact.

31

have high affinity and some will have low affinity. In addition all subclasses of immunoglobulins will be represented amongst the molecules in the serum. This is not the case with monoclonal antibodies. Here only one subclass can be represented with one affinity constant. Many MCA's have low affinity. In the early days of monoclonal antibody production it was thought that monoclonal antibodies had low affinities for biological molecules and would therefore not supersede polyclonal antisera as assay tools. It has now been shown that with adequate selection, high affinity monoclonal antibodies can be made and are reliable tools for immunoassay. For best results the screening of a monoclonal antibody to be used in an assay should be closely linked to the contemplated assay. In this way the antibodies with the most suitable properties will be selected at the start so avoiding disappointment later.

Assay techniques

Standard radioimmunoassay

The usual radioimmunoassay procedure is to take a solution containing the substance to be measured and add to it a standard quantity of radiolabelled similar compound. The antibody is now added, and after a suitable time interval to allow the reaction to occur, the antibody–antigen complex is isolated. The amount of radioactivity present within this is determined on a radioactive counter. The cold antigen present in the sample to be assayed will compete for the radiolabelled antigen added and so if high concentration of cold antigen is present, less radioactivity will bind to the antibody. If only a small amount is present, then the antibody will bind mainly to the radiolabelled antigen and so the precipitate will be highly radioactive (Fig. 3.2).

Immunometric assays

A more rapid and convenient way of performing radioimmunoassays is to use immunometric procedures in a solid phase. This allows rapid, reliable assay under much more standard conditions. There are three methods of performing such immunometric assays each with advantages and disadvantages.

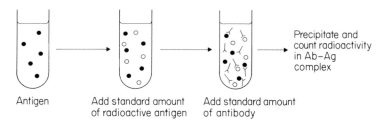

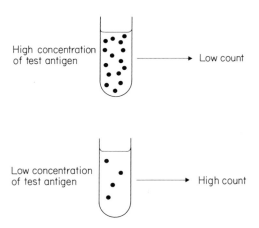

Fig. 3.2. Standard radioimmunoassay where radiolabelled antigen competes for the antibody with the antigen being assayed. The greater the amount of antigen present in the test sample the less the radioactive binding.

The first and most common is the forward-two-step method illustrated in Fig. 3.3. First the antigen is allowed to react with the solid phase absorbent. After an appropriate incubation period, unbound antigen is removed by washing. Radiolabelled antibody then reacts with the bound antigen during the second step. A subsequent buffer wash removes unbound labelled antibody. The label now fixed to the solid phase is directly proportional to the amount of antigen originally in the sample. Monoclonal antibodies used in this forward-two-step assay have a distinct advantage over polyclonal antisera. Absolute specificity provided by the monoclonal antibody means that affinity purification of the antibody is unnecessary.

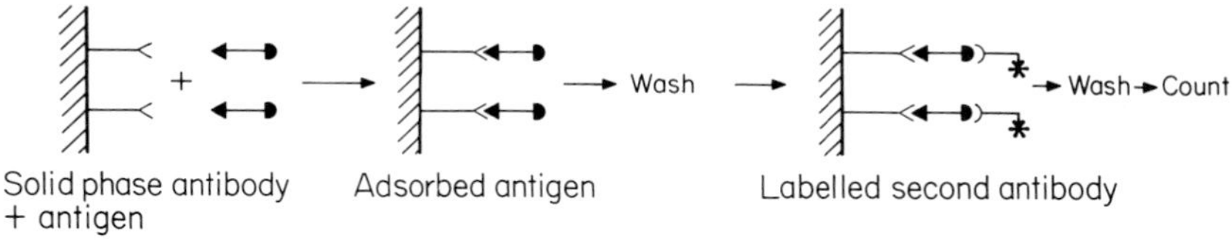

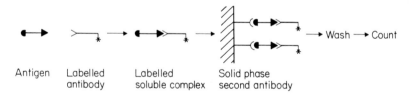

Solid phase antibody + antigen   Adsorbed antigen   Labelled second antibody

Fig. 3.3. Forward-two-step immunometric assay.

The second immunometric assay is the reverse-two-step method. Here the antigen reacts with the labelled antibody in the solution first (Fig. 3.4). After a suitable incubation period the solid phase antibody is added. A wash follows the incubation and again the amount of antigen originally present in the specimen is related to the quantity of label associated with the solid phase. Monoclonal antibodies are distinctly superior in this assay. During the first incubation, a polyclonal antibody will bind most sites in the antigen. A monoclonal antibody on the other hand will bind to a single site and leave the rest of the antigen free to bind to the solid phase.

Antigen   Labelled   Labelled   Solid phase
            antibody   soluble complex   second antibody

Fig. 3.4. Reverse-two-step immunometric assay.

A third type of immunometric assay involves the simultaneous addition of all the reagents and sample together (Fig. 3.5). A single incubation and wash step prepares the solid phase for analysis. This assay works better with monoclonal reagents due to the lack of competition between the binding sites. In addition, the higher capacity of the solid phase to bind MCA delays the saturation effect at extremely high antigen concentrations. This severely limits the use of the low capacity solid phase absorbent made with polyclonal antibodies when used in such assays.

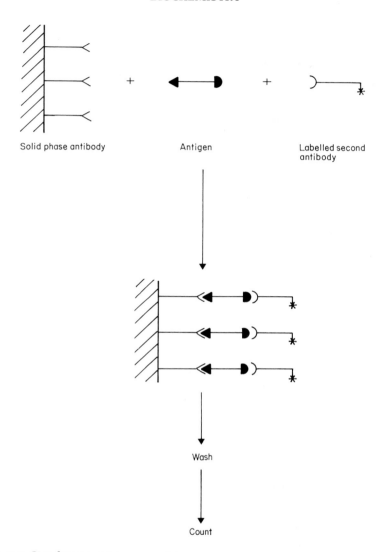

Solid phase antibody   Antigen   Labelled second antibody

Wash

Count

Fig. 3.5. Simultaneous immunometric assay.

Labelled monoclonal antibodies circumvent some of the problems associated with obtaining radiolabelled, purified antigen. It is often difficult to obtain a substance to be assayed in a purified form unless a good assay is already available. It is therefore impossible to obtain a suitable labelled molecule for competition with the antigen present in the sample. Monoclonal antibodies also provide an ideal technique for obtaining antibodies to components in a complex mixture of molecules. If, for example, an animal is immunized with membranes prepared from a tumour cell, a variety of antibodies are made that can be characterized for their specificity. Some may react to blood group substances and to histocompatiblity antigens whilst others may react to molecules expressed in greater quantity on tumour cells than normal cells.

An example of some of the difficulties in assay procedure, where monoclonal antibodies have revolutionized biochemical understanding, is in the analysis of the interferons. Interferon is a protein containing 120 amino acids with a molecular weight of 19,000 daltons. There are several families of interferon which have now been characterized using gene cloning techniques. A major problem until recently was the assay. This previously relied on the inhibition of the viral cytopathic effects described earlier. Before the advent of gene cloning and monoclonal antibodies, it was impossible to obtain any of the interferon family members in a pure form. Many different molecules are present in the stimulated lymphocytes or lymphoblastoid cells used as a source of interferon. By immunizing mice with relatively crude preparations of interferon, monoclonal antibodies were isolated that reacted with single bands of protein on gels. Using these antibodies the proteins were isolated and shown to have defined biological activity. In this way, the circle was closed between the biochemical identification of a molecule and its biological function. In addition, monoclonal antibodies have been useful in the mass production of interferon by gene cloning. Here the DNA sequences coding for interferon are inserted into vectors, which in turn are grown in bacteria, usually *E. coli*. Large quantities of interferon containing supernatant are collected from these bacteria from fermentors such as those used to make wine or beer. There are many bacterial proteins in addition to the interferon present. By using an anti-interferon monoclonal antibody, immobilized on an inert matrix, interferon can be rapidly purified in a continuous process from the fermented supernatant. Although there has been tremendous interest in interferon both in the treatment of infectious diseases and cancer, it remains to be determined whether the expectations will be fulfilled.

Clinical biochemistry

Let us now consider some defined areas in clinical biochemistry where monoclonal antibodies may help over the next few years in the diagnosis and monitoring of various disease states. A major problem in clinical laboratories is the sheer volume of the work load. Using defined reagents many assays can be easily automated, so reducing their cost and making them more widely available.

Heart disease

The heart is one of the most vital organs in the body. A variety of diseases occur in the muscle of the heart which cause the release of intracellular components from damaged heart cells. An example is coronary thrombosis leading to myocardial infarction. Here obstruction occurs in the small coronary blood vessels that supply the heart muscle causing the death of a patch of the myocardium (the muscle block of the heart). The diagnosis of myocardial infarction is not always easy. Although patients may complain of a characteristic type of chest pain, the clinical distinction between various forms of chest pain is often difficult. The use of electrocardiography to identify electrical abnormalities over the heart muscle has proven extremely useful. The measurement of released products by the damaged muscle cells is also extremely useful in the diagnosis of infarction. Enzymes measured include creatinine phosphokinase, oxaloacetate transaminase and pyruvate transaminase. These assays are performed using coloured substrates as described earlier. By developing monoclonal antibodies to these enzymes and to other products that are likely to be released by damaged heart muscle, such as actin and myosin, specific agents can be obtained which can measure the severity of infarction more easily. In addition, by tagging such agents with a radioactive isotope and injecting the antibody intravenously into a patient, a scan can be obtained showing the area of damage. The advent of aggressive surgical techniques to excise damaged myocardium means that such an evaluation is of practical importance in patients being considered for surgery.

Head injury

Another common clinical problem is the assessment of severity of a patient who has had a head injury. Current clinical criteria to assess severity include the clinical history of unconsciousness, amnesia (the period of memory loss), and the presence or absence of a skull fracture. Unfortunately these criteria do not always reflect the severity of internal injury within the brain or the likelihood of late complications, such as intracranial bleeding. Many investigators have made monoclonal antibodies to brain cell proteins, such as creatinine kinase isoenzymes. Such proteins are shed into the serum after head injury. By finding the correct specificity of antibody, precise tools which reflect the severity of cerebral damage may be obtained. This has far reaching implications for the assessment of patients with head injuries. Monoclonal antibodies possess the necessary specificity to distinguish the intracellular products of brain tissue from muscle and liver, organs that are also frequently damaged after accidents.

Cancer

A major problem in treating cancer patients is the inadequate assessment of disease. After primary surgery for breast cancer the chances of small metastases being present, that cannot be detected by currently available techniques, is about 40%. Local treatment of the primary tumour using surgery or radiotherapy is bound to fail to efficiently treat those patients with metastases. If those patients with widespread disease at diagnosis could be identified, aggressive systemic chemotherapy could be used. Similarly, in following patients with lung cancer a small change in the size of the tumour may result in disproportionate changes in the shadow seen on a chest X-ray. This is because tumours in the lung occur in the major bronchi causing obstruction and collapse, with subsequent opacification on a chest X-ray of the lung distal to the tumour. A 1-mm change in tumour diameter could result in complete clearance of opacification seen on a chest X-ray. Several tumours secrete circulating markers that accurately reflect tumour load. These markers include human chorionic gonadotrophins from choriocarcinoma and teratomas; alphafetoprotein from hepatomas and teratomas; immunoglobulins from myelomas; and hormones from hormone-producing tumours. Unfortunately, most of the of common solid tumours, which make up nearly 90% of all cancer, do not have such convenient markers. Monoclonal

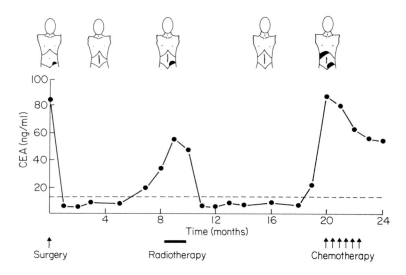

Fig. 3.6. The use of CEA in evaluating disease status in a 62-year-old man with colorectal cancer following surgery.

antibodies may well provide assays for hitherto unknown markers from such tumours.

Colorectal cancer provides an interesting model of how mono-clonal antibodies can increase our ability to measure the disease. On the surface of most colorectal cancers is a complex glycoprotein called carcinoembryonic antigen (CEA). This was discovered by immunizing rabbits with human colon cancer in 1965. The amount of carcinoembryonic antigen shed into the peripheral blood of a patient often reflects accurately the tumour load in an individual patient (Fig. 3.6). Unfortunately, although many trials have been performed using polyclonal antisera to see if the routine assay of CEA could have a place in the diagnosis and management of patients with colorectal cancer, the results have been poor. The reason for this failure is the crossreaction of polyclonal antibodies with a variety of other glyco-proteins, e.g. NCA shed not only by colorectal cancer cells but also normal colon, normal lung epithelium and other normal tissues. Diseases of these structures, or even abnormal life styles such as heavy smoking, result in falsely raised levels of CEA. Monoclonal antibodies allow the fine discrimination of the complex series of molecules that make up the CEA family, making specific identification

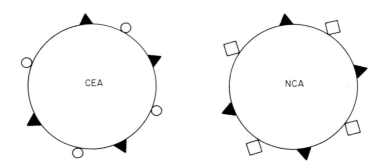

Fig. 3.7. Schematic structure of CEA and NCA.

possible (Fig. 3.7). In this way, more reliable indicators of disease states can be found. Many groups have now produced sets of anti-tumour monoclonal antibodies and are currently evaluating their clinical utility in assays of circulating antigen.

There are limitations to the use of monoclonal antibodies as dis-criminators of tumour load. In measuring CEA, the problem is the heterogeneity of the molecule being assayed. For other molecules this heterogeneity is not a problem. In carcinoma of the prostate the level of acid phosphatase in the peripheral blood is often raised by the out-pouring of the enzyme from neoplastic cells. Serum acid phosphatase provides an indicator of the presence of cancer in a patient with an enlarged prostate. The level of the enzyme also gives information about the size of the tumour and its degree of spread through the body. Unfortunately many patients who have carcinoma of the prostate do not have a significantly raised acid phosphatase. If we look at the distribution of acid phosphatase in the normal population and in the those with carcinoma of the prostate we see there is considerable overlap (Fig. 3.8). Increasing the sensitivity or precision of the assay, will not increase the discrimination between those two populations. However, the availability of a monoclonal reagent, with all its advantages of standardization, allows the development of a cheaper and therefore more widely used assay system.

New assays

The specificity of an MCA makes it an ideal detector reagent in a new breed of ingenious assays. Such assays result in colour changes that

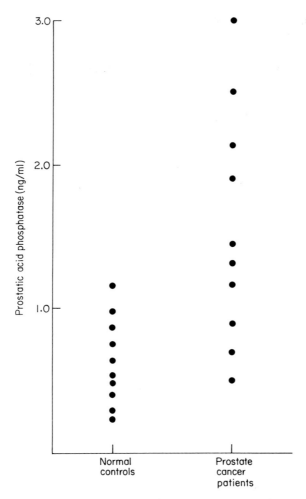

Fig. 3.8. Serum acid phosphatase levels in ten patients with prostate cancer and ten normal controls.

can be read electronically or by the naked eye, in the ward side room. More quantitative determinations can be made using a spectrophotometer. In conventional enzyme-linked immunoabsorbent assay (ELISA) a colourless substrate is converted to a coloured product by the enzyme conjugated to the second antibody. The intensity of this colour is measured directly with a spectrophotometer and is proportional to the concentration of antigen in the original serum sample. In order to develop sufficient colour it is necessary to maximize the amount of enzyme antibody conjugate bound to the solid phase. This usually involves an overnight incubation followed by a lengthy colour development step.

The new amplified enzyme-linked immunoassays follow the ELISA principles up to and including the formation of the antibody/antigen 'sandwich'. Then, however, the activity of the enzyme in the conjugate is not measured directly but is used instead to trigger a secondary, enzyme-mediated colour development process. In this way a small chemical signal is amplified to give an intense colour, easily visible to the naked eye and accurately measurable by machine. The amplifier can have a gain of roughly $500 \times$; each molecule produced by the primary system giving rise to 500 molecules of coloured product during the enzyme-amplified assay. Kits for measuring acid phosphatase by such assays are now commercially available.

Drug assay and overdose

It is possible to make monoclonal antibodies to a wide range of drugs that are used in clinical practice. In this way accurate assays can be developed which allow the true bioavailability of any drug to be determined in an individual. An ingenious use of monoclonal antibodies has recently been described to treat drug overdosage. For certain drugs the difference between a circulating level which is therapeutic and the level which is harmful may be very small. This is due to the variation in the metabolism of the drug by an individual. With certain drugs it is possible for a patient taking a constant daily dose of the drug to accumulate toxic amounts. An example of such a drug is digoxin; a purified glycoside which has many beneficial effects on the heart, strengthening the muscular contractions and slowing the rhythm. It is particularly useful in the treatment of heart failure. Overdosage may easily occur, particularly in elderly patients in whom it is widely prescribed. Such overdosage is characterized by excessive slowing of the pulse, an unpleasant taste in the mouth, nausea, vomiting, blurred vision, convulsions and sometimes death. A reliable assay for the blood level of digoxin helps in finding the exact dose required in an individual patient. Severe overdosage is extremely difficult to treat and up to now no specific therapy has been available. Recently, a study has been reported where a monoclonal antibody was prepared by immunizing animals with digoxin. Anti-digoxin monoclonal antibodies were used to treat patients who showed signs of severe digoxin toxicity. The mechanism of the action is not entirely clear but it appears the antibody was capable of recognizing excess circulating digoxin molecules and causing complexes to be formed which were excreted by the body. All patients treated in this way survived and no untoward effect due to administration of antibody could be identified. This is an extremely encouraging result and there seems to be no reason why such a principle could not be extended to cover other drugs which may be lethal when taken in excess.

Table 3.1.

Biological molecules	Monoclonal antibodies
Surface antigens	Histocompatibility antigens
	Lymphocyte subpopulation antigens
	β_2 microglobulin
	Fibronectin
	Blood group antigens
	Sperm antigens
Proteins	Immunoglobulins
	Glucose-6-phosphate dehydrogenase
	Interferons
	Interleukins
	Fibrinogen
	Complement components
	Blood clotting factors
	Alkaline phosphatase
	Placental acid phosphatase
Tumour markers	Carcinoembryonic antigen
	α-fetoprotein
	β-human chorionic gonadotrophins
	Acid phosphatase
	Oestrogen receptors
Hormones	Somatostatin
	Human growth hormone
	Gastrin
	Oestrogen
	Progesterone

Conclusion

We are now seeing the widespread application of monoclonal anti-bodies in biochemistry. A variety of kits are commercially available for several assays. Table 3.1 lists important biological molecules that can be readily measured using monoclonal antibodies. This list is con-tinually being expanded. Perhaps more importantly monoclonal anti-bodies are providing molecular flags for substances whose true function is yet to be identified.

Further reading

Dale Sevier E., David G.S. & Martinis J. (1981) Monoclonal antibodies in clinical immunology. *Clin. Chem.* **27**, 1797–1806.

McMichael A.J. & Bastin J.M. (1980) Clinical applications of monoclonal anti-bodies. *Immunol. Today*, **2**, 56–61.

Secher D.S. (1981) Immunoradiometric assay of human leukocyte interferon using monoclonal antibody. *Nature*, **290**, 501–503.

Uotila M., Rouoslanti E. & Engvall E. (1981) Two site sandwich enzyme immunoassay with monoclonal antibodies to alpha foetoprotein. *J. Immunol. Methods* **42**, 11–15.

Woodhead J.S., Addison G.M. & Halos C.N. (1974) The immunoradiometric assay and related techniques. *Br. Med. Bull.* **30**, 44–49.

Zola H. (1980) Monoclonal antibodies against the membrane antigens. *Pathology*, **12**, 539–557.

Chapter 4

Histology

PAUL FINAN

The pathological diagnosis of many disease processes rests primarily on the macroscopic appearances of the tissue, followed by careful microscopic examination. The routine use of standard staining techniques, augmented on occasion by stains for specific substances such as amyloid, glycogen, and mucins, provides an accurate diagnosis which then enables the clinician to institute prompt and relevant treatment. Although. these morphological appearances will often suffice, there are occasions when additional information is required. Histological studies using a variety of immunological reagents were, for many years, limited to the interested research worker. However, with improved equipment, more refined techniques and high quality reagents, such studies are rapidly being integrated into general histopathological practice. It is now possible to stain for a wide variety of antigens, hormones, tumour markers, and immunoglobulins which not only enable a diagnosis to be made, but give valuable additional information about the pathogenesis of a particular disease.

Although immunohistological techniques are now generally accepted, a major drawback has been the quality of the reagents used. Conventional polyclonal antisera may contain contaminating immunoglobulins even after extensive absorption. Furthermore, there are often considerable variations in the specificities of antisera obtained from different commercial sources, or from successive bleeds from the same immunized animal. These impurities affect both reliability and reproducibility.

With these limitations in mind it is not surprising that specific, homogenous and well characterized MCA's should rapidly find a place in immunohistology. They offer several advantages with their purity and availability in unlimited quantities, and are likely to replace conventional antisera as standard reagents in the future.

There are already many instances where MCA's have been successfully introduced into histopathological practice, especially in various aspects of cancer diagnosis and research. However, in the first instance, it is worth reviewing the immunohistological techniques that are currently employed.

Immunofluorescence

This technique, introduced in the early 1940s by Coons, relies on a tissue antigen being recognized by an antibody which is coupled to a fluorochrome, usually fluorescein isothiocyanate (FITC). When the tissue section is viewed under ultraviolet light, sites of antigen/antibody interaction may be seen and their tissue distribution recognized. Because conjugation may alter the affinity of an antibody for its antigen, and sampling many individual antibodies for every possible antigen is an exacting task, several indirect or sandwich methods have been introduced. In this way, only a single fluorescent antiglobulin is needed for each animal species. A further advantage to be gained by the indirect technique is one of increased sensitivity. This is due to an amplification of the signal by binding sites on the middle antibody layer acting as antigenic sites for the final fluorochrome-labelled antiglobulin. Such an indirect immunofluorescent technique is outlined diagramatically in Fig. 4.1.

With few exceptions these immunofluorescent techniques have involved the use of frozen tissue sections and although a wide variety of antigens may be demonstrated, there are several disadvantages. The use of frozen sections does not allow retrospective studies, they often give insufficient resolution and the morphological detail is not comparable with paraffin-embedded material. Finally the equipment necessary for reading the result is expensive and this result is not per-manent and so must be recorded on photographic film. For these reasons, several workers have investigated conjugation of the second antibody layer to reagents other than FITC, and in particular, to a variety of enzymes. One such enzyme, horseradish peroxidase (HRP), has been found particularly useful and is being used increasingly in immunohistochemical investigation.

Immunoperoxidase

This method is similar to the fluorescent antibody technique except that conjugation is to the stable enzyme horseradish peroxidase, rather than fluorescein isothiocyanate. Together with hydrogen peroxide, this enzyme polymerizes the substrate diaminobenzidine and results in the formation of an insoluble brown polymer. The advantages of such a method are that the stain is permanent and the

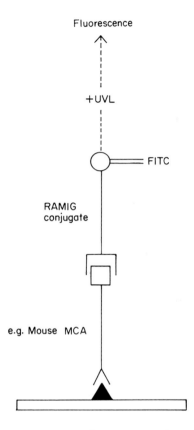

Indirect immunofluorescent technique

Fig. 4.1. Indirect immunofluorescence: a mouse monoclonal antibody
binding to its target antigen. This is detected by rabbit anti-mouse
immunoglobulin (RAMIG) to which FITC (fluorescein isothiocyanate) has
been coupled. Ultraviolet light is directed at the specimen viewed under a
microscope.

section may be suitably counterstained, mounted and viewed under
the standard light microscope. Like the fluorescent techniques, there
are direct and indirect methods, together with more complex sandwich techniques. For comparison the indirect immunoperoxidase
technique is shown diagramatically in Fig. 4.2.

Although fixation and paraffin embedding is likely to destroy some
antigens, it is evident from many reports that a wide variety of tissue

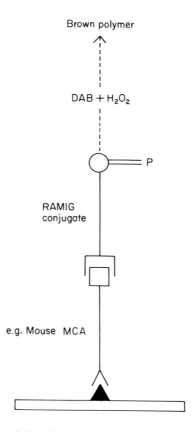

Indirect immunoperoxidase technique

Fig. 4.2. Indirect immunoperoxidase: the same mouse monoclonal antibody is detected by RAMIG conjugated to peroxidase. This enzyme liberates a brown colour in the presence of hydrogen peroxidase (H_2O_2) and diaminobenzidine (DAB).

antigen may be demonstrated in this manner. Furthermore, if a particular antigen is lost in routine fixing, then a variety of other fixatives may be used. The section may also be pretreated by trypsin digestion so unmasking many more cellular antigens.

The ability to detect a particular antigen at a cellular level and at the same time preserve histological detail, is of great value to the histopathologist and with the newer monoclonal reagents there is likely to be a remarkable advance in the understanding of many disease processes. One particular area where monoclonal antibodies have revolutionized histopathological practice is in the field of cancer diagnosis (Plate 1).

Table 4.1 lists some of the clinical advantages to be gained from the immunohistological localization of cellular antigens in malignant tissue. In particular, the detection of various marker substances, e.g. carcinoembryonic antigen, alpha-fetoprotein or human chorionic gonadotrophin might not only assist in the diagnosis of the primary lesion but aid in predicting which substance might be usefully employed in the follow-up period.

Besides these clinical applications, immunohistological studies with monoclonal reagents are being used by many research workers to conduct detailed comparative studies between malignant cell surfaces and their normal counterparts. Such studies are now an integral part of the screening of new monoclonal antibodies with possible clinical potential. In several instances where MCA's were supposed to be detecting an antigen that was restricted to a malignant cell surface alone, and not to the corresponding normal tissue, extensive immunohistological studies have demonstrated the true distribution of the antigen in question. Despite this lack of success in finding 'tumour-specific' MCA's, immunohistological studies have demonstrated other properties of malignant cell surfaces which may

Table 4.1. The value of immunohistological localization of tumour products and antigen

1. Primary diagnosis and differential diagnosis.

2. Suggesting the site of an occult primary lesion by examination of metastatic deposits.

3. Demonstration of small foci of tumour not readily seen with conventional stain.

4. Discrimination between tumours which appear similar using conventional histological criteria.

5. Determines the site within tumour cell responsible for marker substance production.

6. Determines the most useful marker substances with which to monitor patient.

be of value in the future. In several cases, heterogeneity of antigenic expression of morphologically similar cells has been demonstrated and such a finding may account for the observed variation in response to treatment of apparently similar tumours. In addition, it has been shown that even normally occurring antigens may be lost from tumour cell surfaces and that this may have additional prognostic significance. Besides the continued use of immunohistological methods by research workers, there are now many reports of the successful incorporation of MCA's into general histopathological practice.

A set of MCA's has been made against human lymphocytes and is called the OKT series. These antibodies define antigen expression at different stages of maturation of the human T-lymphocytes (cf. Chapter 6). OKT9 and OKT10 recognize antigens present on immature thymocytes which during maturation are gradually lost and replaced with a cell surface antigen more characteristic of the mature cell, recognized by OKT3. Using a panel of the OKT series, cells from patients with lymphocytic leukaemia have been analysed. It seems likely that with further use, these reagents will not only assist in classifying leukaemia but also in predicting the probable clinical course of individual patients. Children with T-cell acute lymphoblastic leukaemia comprising the 'suppressor' subset of T-lymphocytes (reacting with OKT8) fare better than those with similar disorders derived from the 'helper' subset (recognized by OKT4). One further aspect revealed in such studies has been the diversity in antigen expression within apparently similar tumours. Mycosis fungoides, a cutaneous T-cell lymphoma, has been shown to be derived from the 'helper' T-cell subset of lymphocytes and to be fairly homogenous in its expression of the surface antigen T_4. In contradistinction patients with T-cell lymphoblastic lymphoma show considerable heterogeneity within their tumours.

The distinction between non-Hodgkin's lymphoma and undifferentiated tumours of non-haemopoeitic origin may be difficult, on purely morphological grounds, under the light microscope. A MCA, T29/33, which stains only the tumours of lymphoid origin has successfully distinguished these tumours in 150 cases (40 lymphomas and 110 selected and representative tumours of non-haemopoeitic tissue). Panels of MCA's have been used in difficult cases and the pattern of activity suggested the type of malignant tumour present. Similarly, as more MCA's are characterized then the histopathologist will be able to distinguish between different types of tumour from the same organ. For example, a set of antibodies which differentiate small cell, adenocarcinoma and squamous carcinomas of the lung from bronchio-alveolar or large cell lung cancers has now been produced.

Frequently the pathologist is faced with a small specimen on which to make a diagnosis, these being obtained by needle biopsy, fine needle aspiration or examination of an effusion or ascites. There is evidence that MCA's will allow more rapid diagnosis of the underlying malignancy. Lymphoblastic disorders in children can be rapidly distinguished using a panel of thirteen MCA's. Similarly two MCA's, HMFG2 and AKAI, directed to epithelial cell determinants, were able to detect malignant cells in serous effusions. Both antibodies fail to react with non-epithelial, mesothelial and endothelial cells, so distin-guishing cancer cells in pleural and peritoneal fluid.

The recognition of small foci of malignant cells, not immediately apparent on routine examination, is of obvious prognostic importance when examining various tissue, e.g. bone marrow and lymph nodes. The value of immunohistological studies on these tissues has already been mentioned and will be greatly facilitated with the increasing number of MCA's that are becoming commercially available.

Although as yet no truly tumour-specific antigen has been demon-strated, there are many substances which, because of extraordinary quantitative differences between normal and malignant tissue, can act as tumour markers. Their particular importance is in the follow-up of the treated patient. Examples include alpha-fetoprotein in teratomas and hepatomas, human chorionic gonadotrophin in chorio-carcinoma and carcinoembryonic antigen in several epithelial tumours, particularly those of gastrointestinal origin. The most valuable marker substance in an individual tumour might be predicted by immunohistological studies of the resected tissue and MCA's have been produced to many of these markers.

Conclusion

Although the monoclonal antibody technology is still in its infancy the availability of large quantities of well characterized, pure and homo-genous reagents has revolutionized the immunohistological examina-tion of normal and malignant tissues. These techniques have aided in the diagnosis and classification of tumours. They have also demonstrated, in many instances, heterogeneity within tumours which may well account for differences in response to treatment. It seems likely that in the not too distant future, similar studies will shed light on many of the problems that have bedevilled researchers and clinicians alike.

Further reading

Burns J. (1978) Immunohistological methods and their application in the routine laboratory. In *Recent Advances in Histopathology* (Eds P.P. Anthony & N. Woolf), pp. 337–349. Churchill Livingstone, Edinburgh.

De Lellis R.A., Sternberger L.A., Mann R.B., Banks P.M. & Nakene P.K. (1979) Immunoperoxidase techniques in diagnostic pathology. *Am. J. Clin. Pathol.* **71**, 483–488.

Epenetos A.A., Canti G., Taylor-Papadimitriou J., Gurling M. & Bodmer W.F. (1982) Use of two epithelial-specific monoclonal antibodies for diagnosis of malignancy in serous effusion. *Lancet*, **ii**, 1004–1006.

Finan P.J., Grant R.M., de Mattos C.M., Takei F., Berry J.M., Lennox E.S. & Bleehen N.M. (1982) The use of immunohistological techniques as an aid in th early screening of monoclonal antibodies. *Br. J. Cancer* (1982) **46**, 9–17.

Heyderman E. (1979) Immunoperoxidase technique in histopathology: applications, methods and controls. *J. Clin. Pathol.* **32**, 971–978.

Kemshead J.T., Goldman A., Fritschy J., Malpas J.G. & Pritchard J. (1983) Use of panels of monoclonal antibodies in the differential diagnosis of neuroblastoma and lymphoblastic disorders. *Lancet*, **i**, 12–15.

Naiem M., Gerder J., Abdullaziz Z., Sunderland C.A., Allington M.J., Stein H. & Mason D.Y. (1982) The value of immunohistological screening in the production of monoclonal antibodies. *J. Immunol. Methods*, **50**, 145–160.

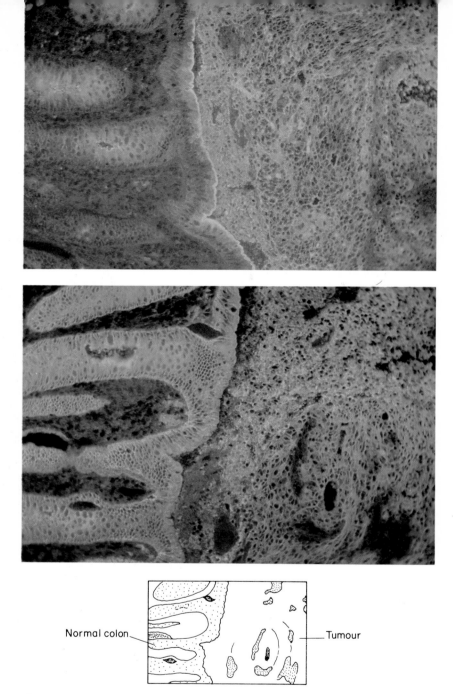

Normal colon — ⟨diagram⟩ — Tumour

Plate 1   Sections of normal and malignant colon stained using indirect
immunofluorescence with two different MCA's raised by immunizing rats
with fresh colorectal cancer cells. The top shows selectivity of the antibody
for the tumour whilst the bottom does not.

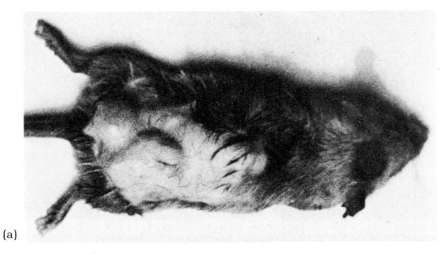

(a)

Plate 2   Radiolabelled MCA administration to a mouse bearing a human colon carcinoma. (a) Mouse bearing carcinoma above right leg; (b) blood pool image using ^{99M}Tc as described in Chapter 8; (c) ^{131}I-labelled MCA scan; (d) subtraction of image (b) from (c) showing tumour outline. The red areas have the highest uptake of isotope.

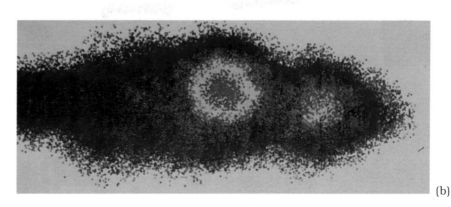

(b)

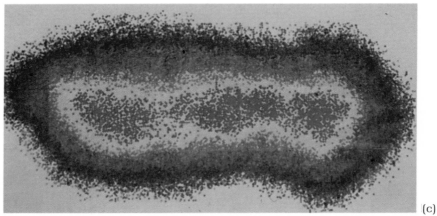

(c)

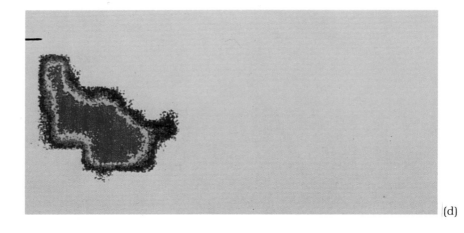

(d)

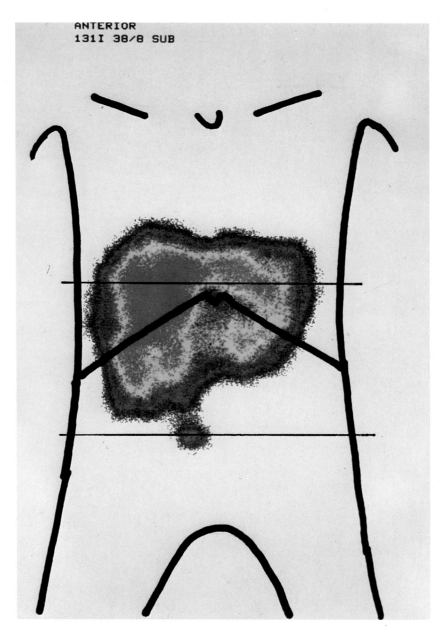

Plate 3   A 16-year-old girl with extensive liver replacement by hepatoma.
On scanning with a radiolabelled MCA the tumour deposits in the liver are
outlined as well as a deposit of tumour in the right para-aortic nodal area.
This distribution of tumour is confirmed by CT scanning at the level of the
liver (top) and para-aortic mass (bottom).

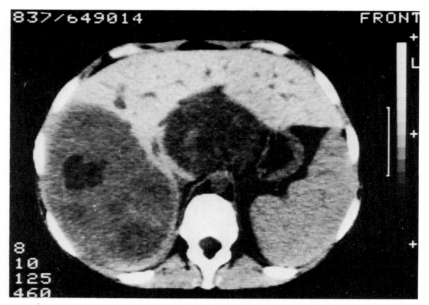

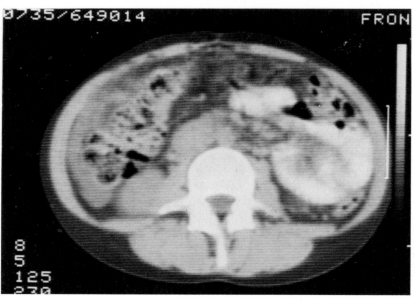

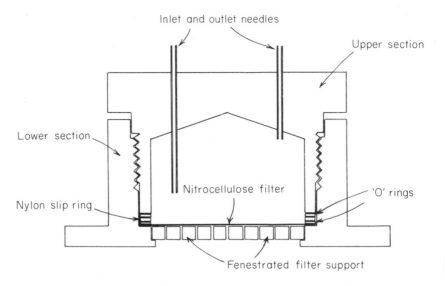

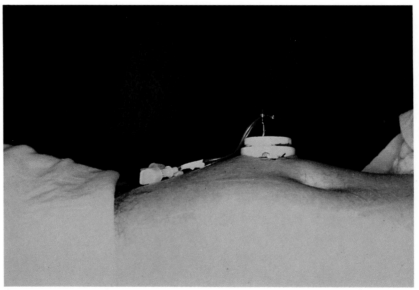

Plate 4 A subcutaneous chamber in which hybridoma cells can grow. The top diagram shows the construction method and the bottom picture, the chamber inserted in the anterior abdominal wall of a patient.

Chapter 5

Microbiology

A micro-organism is a living creature too small to visualize with the naked eye. Medical microbiology is the study of the role of micro-organisms in health and in disease. The first description of micro-organisms comes from Anthony van Leuwenhoek, who observed minute living creatures in pond water in 1674. Most of the early observations and experimental work were performed with bacteria and until comparatively recently the terms microbiology and bacteriology were considered synonymous. It is now clear that bacteria are only one of a number of types of organisms responsible for disease. Viruses, fungi, protozoa and helminths are all important pathogens.

Except for the neonate, within the first hours of life, the human body lives in a state of symbiosis with many different types of micro-organisms. It is normal, and indeed beneficial, to have micro-organisms inhabiting the alimentary tract and these bacteria play a vital role in the metabolism and excretion of certain body compounds, e.g. bilirubin. In health, micro-organisms may also be found in skin, the female genital tract, the urinary tract and the upper air passages. Disease resulting from micro-organisms occurs due to one of three mechanisms.

1 Organisms which are normally present in small quantities suddenly show unrestrained growth in either their normal location or in an area where they are not normally encountered. For example, patients who are immunosuppressed from prolonged corticosteroid ingestion may develop a gross oral infection with *Candida albicans*, the clinical condition known as thrush. This is caused by a yeast normally found in small amounts as a commensal in mucous membranes.

2 If the normal defence mechanisms, such as the anatomical barriers or immune defence systems of the host, are deficient in any way organisms normally foreign to the host may enter and cause disease. The most common example of this occurs after injury where

the normal protective barrier of the host, the skin, is damaged and access may be afforded to various organisms so causing systemic disease. In patients with deep penetrating wounds, which are inadequately cleaned, the anaerobic bacteria *Clostridium welchii* may gain access and find the abnormal conditions suitable for its growth and therefore colonize the host causing gas gangrene.

3   Infectious diseases are those diseases in which the passage of a causative organism from one person to the next is responsible for the transmission of the disease. Such organisms may be viruses, bacteria or protozoa. Probably the best example is the common cold which is caused by a rhinovirus transmitted in droplets, especially during sneezing and coughing, and so is widely contagious. Other routes of transmission are recognized and Table 5.1 gives a list of the known methods of transmission of disease.

Once a micro-organism has gained access to the host, the host's immune response is paramount in determining the outcome of that particular infection and the response of the host to subsequent re-infection with the same or similar organisms. Let us consider the case of a simple bacterial infection of the skin. If, following a wound, an infecting organism gains access to the host then a non-specific inflammatory response will ensue. This will cause the skin around the wound to become hot, swollen, red and tender. This is the body's attempt to seal off an area of injury. Macrophages are activated which destroy the invader. Specific immune responses are also evident, coating the pathogen with antibody so making it easily recognizable for destruction. If the immune response of the host is competent then the wound, with the surrounding area, will be effectively sealed off by the host and as the dead tissue and invading organisms are destroyed pus

Table 5.1. Routes of transmission and some common examples

Routes	Examples
Direct Contact	Gonorrhoea
Fomites	Ringworm
Air	Influenza
Dust	Tuberculosis
Insects	Malaria
Water	Cholera
Food	Staphylococcus
Soil	Clostridium species

will form which may lead to abscess formation. Should the invading micro-organisms gain access into the patient's blood circulation then systemic symptoms will ensue. These take the form of fever, sweating, general malaise and headache. The presence in the blood stream of bacteria at this time is called a bacteraemia and in the presence of clinical symptoms the patient is said to have septicaemia. In the pre-antibiotic days no specific therapy was available. Either the patient was able to produce antibodies to the responsible organism after a period of 7 to 14 days which destroyed the pathogen, the fever would 'break' and the patient would slowly recover or if the patient was unable to manufacture adequate antibody then his condition would deteriorate and he would die. Such an outcome is still occasionally encountered today when the patient has a grossly deficient immune system, as with long-term immunosuppressive therapy after kidney transplantation or if inappropriate antibiotic therapy is given.

It may be that the organism responsible for infection, is capable of inducing a strong antibody reaction if lymphocytes have been 'primed' to recognize a particular antigen on the micro-organism and the immune memory of the patient will result in the rapid production of specific antibodies. This is widely seen in the common childhood ill-nesses such as rubella where a second infection in a normal healthy patient is exceedingly rare.

Immunization

The other aspect of medical practice in which an understanding of the immunology of micro-organisms is important is in prevention. Immunization is either 'active' or 'passive'. In active immunization a vaccine is administered to the patient which contains micro-organisms which are antigenically identical to those capable of causing a disease. This is done either by taking a virulent organism and killing it, usually by heating, prior to inoculation so that the organism is antigenically intact but incapable of self-multiplication. Alternatively a live attenuated organism is administered; this is an organism which is identical to that capable of causing disease but is sufficiently different to be harmless to the patient. In this way, the patient's immune system can recognize and manufacture antibodies to each of the antigenic determinants on the organism and therefore be protected from subsequent re-infection from the virulent counter-

part. In passive immunization, the patient is given antibodies manufactured outside the body capable of recognizing and destroying
infectious organisms. Such antisera are made in horses or other
animals and are only given to patients who are already infected with
an organism likely to cause disease for which there is no specific
therapy. Passive immunization by the administration of animal
immunoglobulin is fraught with problems for the clinician and the
patient and the prospect of monoclonal antibodies produces much
hope for improvement here, as in other areas of medical microbiology.

There are several areas in which monoclonal antibodies promise
to result in significant advances in our understanding of the biology
and therapy of infectious diseases. These may be considered under
four headings.

1   Diagnosis of infectious diseases.
2   Classification of micro-organisms.
3   Immunization.
4   Understanding the ultra-structure of micro-organisms.

Diagnosis of infectious disease

When a physician is faced with a patient suffering from an infectious
disease it is essential that he is able to obtain a rapid and accurate
diagnosis in order to be able to offer the patient the best possible treatment. Although in certain bacterial infections antibiotic therapy has
been the major success of recent years, the same cannot be said of
infections with viruses and some other organisms. In addition, the
emergence of antibiotic resistant bacteria make it likely that
increasing efforts must be made to produce more specific therapies,
for example targeting of otherwise toxic molecules to a desired end-
point. At present diagnosis is usually done by one of the following
methods:

1   Direct microscopic examination of clinical material hoping to
recognize the morphology of bacteria, fungi, parasites or certain
virus-infected cells. Although this can be successful if the responsible
organism is seen, this may not be possible and is therefore only helpful
in a limited number of cases.

2   Culture; involving the use of different growth media to provide the
conditions in which pathogenic organisms may multiply better than
normal commensals and so permit identification by a combination of

microscopy and chemical analysis. This is an extremely time-consuming and labour intensive operation, which even under optimal circumstances will take several days to produce a definitive answer for the clinician. In many cases this delay is too long.

3   Serological tests to identify the presence of antigens within the patient associated with a certain disease, e.g. HBsAg which is found in patients suffering from hepatitis B.

4   The measurement of specific antibodies produced by the host in response to the presence of the infecting organism. With the relatively insensitive polyclonal antibody analysis performed at present it is usually not possible to detect the presence of active infection, except in certain rare disorders. More commonly it is found that the patient has a low titre of antibody to a certain organism which indicates that the disease is either present or has been present at some point in the past. Only if the concentration of such an antibody rises with time is it possible to identify the exact cause of an infection. This is often the case in certain rickettsial disorders where so-called acute and convalescent sera are taken to monitor the changing titre of antibodies to a panel of infecting organisms. In this instance the diagnosis is often retrospective and may not help the clinician treating an acute episode. Clearly the role of monoclonal antibody technology, to produce more specific and rapid diagnosis, is of immense importance.

To take a simple example, if we consider the outer surface of an organism such as a bacterium then it is obvious that, antigenically, such a surface is extremely complex. Many thousands or millions of epitopes are present, each capable of giving rise to an antibody. The difference between different species or subspecies may be extremely small and too subtle for unravelling by conventional polyclonal antibodies. As we have frequently said before, monoclonal antibodies have great specificity, react with uniform affinity, can be produced in endless quantities and purified to homogeneity relatively easily. By using whole organisms as the immunogen and extensive screening of the hybrids produced, species-specific antibodies may be discovered. Unfortunately, such a simple distinction may not be found. Antigenic differences may arise by possession of unique permutations of several antigens, which in turn can be recognized by different MCA's. In this case, rapid diagnosis may be made by using a panel of monoclonal antibodies, each recognizing a specific antigen.

Sexually transmitted diseases

Such a system as already been described looking at the application of MCA's to the diagnosis of sexually transmitted diseases. In these conditions it is important for the clinician to be able to distinguish between different types of organisms, which may produce identical clinical pictures, e.g. *Neisseria gonorrhoea*, *Chlamydia genitalis* and *Herpes simplex* type 2. Not only is this distinction important but different species of the Neisseria genus may also differ in their sensitivity to treatment. By using conventional methods of diagnosis it may take up to 7 days to reach a definitive microbiological answer. In practice the situation is even more complex in that these organisms may be co-transmitted; for example, 20% of heterosexual males and 40% of heterosexual females with gonorrhoea are also infected with Chlamydia. A panel of antibodies has been produced by immunization with *Neisseria gonorrhoea*. Following screening, it was not possible to detect an antibody which was capable of recognizing *N. gonorrhoea* without cross reaction to other Neisseria species. However a panel of sixteen monoclonal antibodies was screened and it was found that each antibody reacted with a characteristic subset of bacteria. Further *in vitro* work enabled the identification of the antigen recognized by each antibody; three monoclonal antibodies were pooled and specific reaction patterns with *Neisseria gonorrhoea* were found in 99.6% of the samples studied.

Exciting results have been reported using a fluorescein conjugated MCA to produce immunofluorescent staining of cultured specimens to diagnose *Chlamydia genitalis*. At present, conventional diagnostic methods require 72–96 hr of culture followed by iodine staining and light microscopy to demonstrate the presence of viral inclusion bodies. The use of immunofluorescence employing an antibody prepared against a major membrane protein of Chlamydia showed that the sensitivity of this new method was at least four times greater than the conventional method and a direct examination could be made which may take less than 30 min to perform in the clinic. Such rapid and reliable diagnosis would represent an advance in the diagnosis of the sexually transmitted diseases.

Tuberculosis

Another aspect of bacteriology, where monoclonal antibodies have been used to advantage, is in the diagnosis of tuberculosis. Tuber-culosis is still a very common disease world-wide, especially in the Third World countries. The disease in man may be caused by several species of mycobacteria. Strains exist of each species which are known to be antigenically different in different parts of the world. The use of monoclonal antibodies which recognize unique epitopes, on different strains of each species, can be used to make rapid and accurate diagnosis. Of especial value would be the accurate diagnosis of active infection. So many people world-wide receive immunization BCG at an early age, that it is common for a positive reaction to the skin testing to be found. This is difficult to interpret as it may indicate the presence of active disease but may also mean that the patient has been exposed to the tubercle bacillus in the past. Therefore, the diagnosis of active infection can be difficult and often requires complex biological assays of clinical specimens in live animals, such as guinea-pigs, to see if they develop the clinical disease. This test may take six weeks in order to produce a result. A panel of antibodies each recognizing a different type or form of the infecting organism would be useful in producing an answer to this vexing clinical problem.

Parasitology

A parasite is an organism which is dependant for its existence on living inside or outside another organism. Parasites may be symbiotic, i.e. they may be harmless to the host or even provide some benefit, in return for a favourable environment in which to live. In medical prac-tice, parasites are those organisms which cause harm. On a global scale most of the diseases caused to man result from parasitic infec-tion, and in addition they are a cause of much morbidity amongst animals, which in turn has consequences for human nutrition.

Because of the diversity of these organisms it follows that they have relatively complex life cycles. That is to say at different points of their evolution, they exist in different morphological forms and inhabit different environments. Many parasites have a life cycle outside man; for example the malaria-causing family Plasmodii, also live in mosquitoes. Similarly the tape worm *Taeniae coli*, which is a cause of malabsorption in man, also lives in the muscle of pigs. By inference, therefore, just as the parasite may alter its morphological form, it follows that its antigenic constitution is likely to alter dramatically during the life cycle. The implications of this are enormous.

Firstly, the host will only be able to develop antibodies to certain stages of the life cycle, and this may be important in developing resistance. The host will produce antibodies against the parasites which may be specific to a stage of development, i.e. stage specific, and which may also be specific to particular strains of an infecting organism in conditions where several strains or species may be responsible for the same disease. In the case of malaria, for example, even individuals who have had the disease may readily become re-infected if chemical prophylaxis is discontinued whilst the patient is in an area of high endemic activity. Figure 5.1 gives a diagrammatic representation of the natural history of malaria in mosquitoes and man. From this we can see that the disease has several cycles which include inoculation of the sporozoites by the mosquito, followed by merozoite infection of the liver, and a red blood cell phase with schizonts which rupture, with periodicity characteristic of the disease. There are reports of monoclonal antibodies being raised against the sporozoite phase of the disease, which may protect the host from subsequent infection when challenged with further sporozoite inoculation. Antibodies against specific blood-stage antigens raise the possibility of an effective vaccine against malaria in

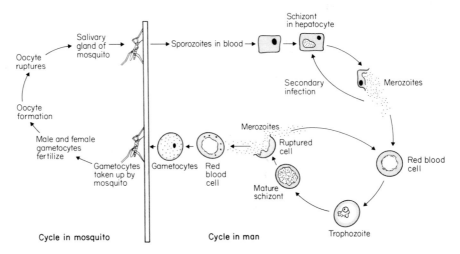

Fig. 5.1. The life cycle of plasmodium, the causative organism of malaria, showing its different forms.

man. Certainly work already performed has done much to characterize these stage-specific antigens and promises useful results at least in the species studied. Although this work is at an early stage, it is clear that monoclonal antibody technology has provided a useful tool with which to explore in depth the antigenic ultra-structure of the malaria parasite and suggest methods of overcoming clinical disease.

Immunization

Immunization means acquiring protection against a disease. Effectively this means giving a patient antibodies or the ability to produce antibodies against antigens found on a particular pathogen. Active immunization by vaccination is well established and highly effective in many common diseases and in combination with public health measures has led to the total eradication of certain diseases, e.g. smallpox. The question of passive immunization however is more problematical. Antibodies need to be given to patients in several situations:

1   Where the patient's immune system is compromised, either due to immunodeficiency or immunosuppression. In these situations the patient is unable to manufacture antibodies even when challenged by a pathogenic organism.

2   In certain virulent disorders, such as rabies, the natural history of the disease, following infection of the host is so rapid that death will occur before the patient has had time to mount an immune response.

3   Active immunization involves the use of live vaccines. In these circumstances the organism chosen is normally a live avirulent or a harmless variant of the organism which causes the disease. When vaccinated with such an organism the patient may have mild systemic symptoms such as fever for a few days, or even develop a very mild form of the disease, but in doing so acquires protection against the more serious and life-threatening organisms. An example of such reaction is the variola-minor reaction sometimes seen after smallpox injections. In people with inadequate immune defence systems, even the use of such mild vaccines may be associated with a significant form of the disease. For example, in children undergoing chemotherapy for acute leukaemias, who come into contact with diseases such as chickenpox, it may be necessary to administer prepared immunoglobulin.

In nearly all the above cases, the so-called 'immune serum' or anti-serum is obtained from injecting immunocompetent animals with the offending organism and then obtaining and purifying serum from these animals to inject into the patient. The horse was frequently used for this purpose in the past as large amounts of serum could be obtained over a long period, without detriment to the health of the animal. However, whatever purification method is used the patient receives foreign proteins from another species. This may lead to an unwanted allergic reaction, causing serum sickness which in itself can be a life-threatening condition. Monoclonal antibodies offer several advantages.

Firstly, it is possible to produce antibodies of a very high speci-ficity which can be used in passive immunization. An attractive pro-position would be the production of hybrids, using human lymphocytes fused with a human myeloma line, to produce antibodies against a specified pathogenic antigen. Although human–human fusions tend to have low rates of immunoglobulin secretion, it should be possible to have hybrid cultures constantly available, producing immunoglobulin which could be purified and stored so that adequate amounts are available for clinical usage (cf. Chapter 10).

In other special circumstances there would be advantages in intro-ducing the hybrid cells into the patient directly by means of a subcuta-neous chamber. This device, which is further described in Chapter 10, enables the hybridoma cells to live for long periods of time when inserted into the patient's subcutaneous tissue, in such a way that a membrane filter prevents the passage of hybridoma cells into the patient's systemic circulation, but allows free diffusion of nutrients into the chamber and free diffusion of immunoglobulin out of the chamber. In this way constant amounts of immunoglobulin are secreted into the patient's circulation. This would allow adequate pro-tection over long periods of time. As the human–human fusion is producing a human protein, no cross species allergic reactions could occur. The relative safety of injection of large amounts of human monoclonal antibodies, produced in this way, has already been established in experiments using human monoclonal antibodies for use in scanning in patients with malignant disease.

Virology

Viruses are amongst the simplest biological structures known. At their very simplest, they consist of a small nucleic acid core, known as the genome, approximately 25–30 nm in diameter and a surrounding protein coat, known as the capsid. The nucleic acid is either RNA or DNA, but not both. These viruses are obligatory intracellular parasites and divide by replication inside the host cell, which is converted into a virus production unit. In man the main defences against viruses are primary and non-specific immune mechanisms. Clinical infections may pass before circulating antibodies can be produced against the infecting organism, although cell-mediated immunity is obviously important in developing memory to previous viral infections.

At present the mainstay of diagnosis is by serology using conventional complement fixation and haemagglutination techniques, many of which require paired samples — that is to say, serum obtained at the time of acute infection and at subsequent times. The diagnosis may only be made by measuring the change in concentration of certain classes of antibodies. This is obviously of limited practical value to the clinician treating a patient with an acute illness as the time required for accurate diagnosis is often weeks or months. Monoclonal antibodies will make a unique contribution in the diagnosis of viral illnesses.

Although many viruses have a stable antigenic complement and thus allow the development of an immune memory, there is a phenomenon known as antigenic drift, best seen in the influenza viruses where the type and distribution of antigens is constantly changing. This explains the observation that a patient may exhibit no resistance to infection with a virus relatively soon after a previous infection. The shift of antigenic structure has prevented the development of an adequate immunological memory. By using these antibodies it is now possible to perform structural analysis of the influenza virus and catalogue in a detailed fashion the frequency of different variants. The influenza virus genus comprises of two viruses, type A and type B, which have no crossreaction with each other. Of the A species, subtypes are recognized which differ in their haemagglutin (HA) and neuraminidase (NA) antigens, but share a type-specific nucleoprotein (NP) and other antigens. As a result of the antibodies recognizing different epitopes on the HA antigen, it is possible to see how changes in the structure of the single molecule result in many different strains of the influenza A virus and suggests that the evolution of new species is caused by a high frequency of point mutation causing a major antigenic change. Extrapolating this type of work, it is now possible to perform sophisticated epidemiological surveys of the patterns of spread and distribution of viral epidemics. It is also clear that certain strains of virus arise which have previously been encountered. Similar studies have been performed for the proteins of rabies and rabies-related viruses.

When the question of diagnosis is considered, in relation to viral diseases, the very nature of the specificity of monoclonal antibodies may be a disadvantage. Many viruses vary in antigenic structure and natural variation in characteristic epitopes means that monoclonal antibodies of high specificity may fail to recognize a common antigen. Under these circumstances, it would seem advisable to use a panel of monoclonal antibodies in order to recognize patterns rather than rely on single antibodies. Monoclonal antibodies have already been found useful in the fluorescent antibody staining of brain smears from animals infected with rabies and some work had been reported using monoclonal antibodies to detect the surface antigen in hepatitis B.

Another exciting aspect of virology is the possible development of vaccine against certain virus-induced conditions. The Epstein–Barr (EB) virus is a human herpes virus whose target cells are primarily the B-lymphocyte line. The EB virus is widely distributed in all human communities and is known to be reponsible for infectious mononucleosis in adolescents. However this virus has also been associated with two human malignancies, Burkitt's lymphoma — a malignant condition of childhood mainly found in Africa — and in poorly differentiated nasopharyngeal carcinoma. Extensive work done on Burkitt's lymphoma shows that patients with this condition have high levels of antibodies to the virus capsid antigen and that the tumour cells from these patients all carry the EB virus genome. Other epidemiological evidence also supports this conclusion. However, co-factors are clearly important in the development of this condition, which is found in a narrow geographical area compared to the world-wide distribution of the EB virus. It would appear that endemic malaria is the important factor.

The evidence for the involvement of EB virus with nasopharyngeal carcinoma is similar. In this malignancy the known co-factors include racial predisposition, and the possession of histocompatibility types HLA A2 and BW46. Several different types of antigen are known to be associated with the presence of EB virus within a cell. These EB-virus-induced antigens can be found within the nucleus, the cytoplasm and on the membrane of infected cells. It is already possible to produce monoclonal antibodies to many of the EB-virus-induced membrane antigens. This gives rise to the hope that it may be possible to develop vaccines which could stimulate the host to recognize and respond to EB-virus-induced antigens and thus protect the host from the development of these aggressive malignancies.

Further reading

Cohen S. (1982) Immunology of Malaria. In: *Clinical Aspects of Immunology* (Eds P.J. Lachmann & D.K. Peters) 5th ed. Blackwell Scientific Publications, Oxford.

Gerhard W., Yewdell J., Frankel M., Lopes A. & Staudt L. (1980) Monoclonal antibodies against influenza virus. In: *Monoclonal Antibodies* (Eds R.H. Kennett, T.J. McKearn & K.B. Bechtol). Plenum Press, New York.

McMichael A.J. & Fabre J.W. (1982) *Monoclonal Antibodies in Clinical Medicine*. Academic Press, London.

Nowinski R.C., Tam M., Goldstein L.C., Stone L., Kuo C.C., Corey L., Stamm W.E., Handsfield H. & Knapp J.S. (1982) Monoclonal antibodies for diagnosis of infectious diseases in humans. *Science*, **219**, 637–644.

Sursman M. (1982) Diagnosis of bacterial disease. In: *Clinical Aspects of Immunology*. (Eds P.J. Lachmann & D.K. Peters) 5th ed. Blackwell Scientific Publications, Oxford.

Chapter 6

Haematology

Many disorders can affect the production and function of blood cells. Haematology is an important clinical discipline requiring precise assays. Much of the work of the clinical haematology laboratory is automated; red and white cells can be counted by their ability to produce electrical impulses when flowing between two electrodes. Counters which work on this principle provide the rapid assessment of the number and type of cells found in the blood stream. Blood transfusion is an important procedure in modern medicine as blood is lost not only after accidental injury and in childbirth but also during most major surgical procedures. Its controlled replacement prevents the development of shock with subsequent deleterious consequences. Red cells have numerous inherited antigens on their surface which induce antibodies if given to a person who does not express the same antigens on his or her red cells. The work of the blood transfusion laboratory is to type red cells so ensuring that transfusions are compatible. In addition, there is a lethal but preventable disease (haemolytic disease of the newborn) which occurs in the developing fetus of rhesus-negative pregnant women who have children by rhesus-positive men. This is caused by the haemolysis of red cells by anti-rhesus antibodies. Correct determination of the blood group of the mother, and if necessary the fetus, is possible using serological techniques. Haematology also includes the study of blood clotting — a complex process which involves circulating platelets in the peripheral blood, together with a variety of serum proteins which interact to form a cascade (Fig. 6.1). This cascade results in the conversion of fibrinogen to fibrin and the formation of a blood clot. A second system is available to dissolve the clot — the plasminogen plasmin system. Several diseases are caused or exacerbated by disorders of clotting. To study the reasons for these disorders we need clearly defined assays for the various factors involved.

Monoclonal antibodies have now had an impact in all these areas. Over the next decade we will see the routine application of monoclonal antibodies in transfusion laboratories. At present 90% of blood group determinations performed in the U.K. are already carried out

66

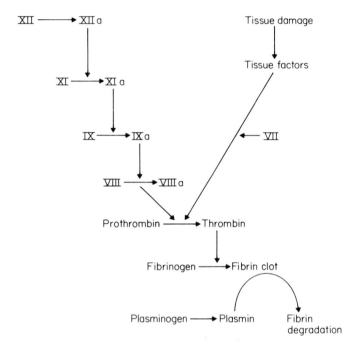

Fig. 6.1. The blood clotting system. A complex cascade of factors (Roman numerals) that when activated result in the formation of a fibrin clot. These factors can now be identified by MCA's.

using commercially produced monoclonal anti-A and anti-B blood grouping reagents.

Blood transfusion

Red cells are involved in the carriage of oxygen from the lungs to the tissues, and possess highly immunogenic structures on their surface (Fig. 6.2). These antigens are determined by a complex molecular display pattern, produced by the sequence and spatial arrangement of sugar molecules in glycolipids and glycoproteins, on their external surface. The antigens were recognized when blood transfusion was

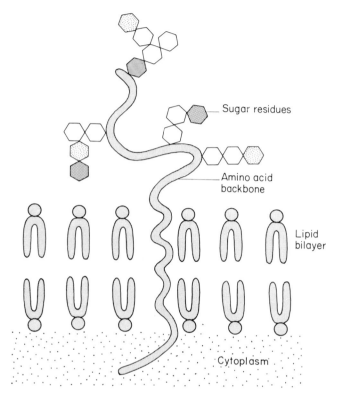

Fig. 6.2. Schematic diagram of transmembrane molecules of red blood cells bearing sugar residues. These glycoproteins can be specifically recognized by MCA's.

performed. Some patients were found to lyse the donor red cells. Further studies showed that this lysis could be predicted by taking serum from a patient and mixing it with donor red cells prior to transfusion. If the cells clumped together, a process called agglutination, then a transfusion reaction was likely.

Let us consider the simple ABO blood group system. The ABO antigens are immunodominant molecules present on all human red cells. The precursor molecule is termed H. The subsequent modification of the carbohydrate grouping on H is genetically determined. In about one third of the population no change occurs, neither blood group A nor B is found. Such patients are group 'O'. However, in other members of the population genes code for a series of enzymes, the

Table 6.1.

Antigens	Genotype	Natural antibodies
O	OO	anti A,B
A	AA or AO	anti B
B	BB or BO	anti A
AB	AB	none

glycosyl transferases, to change the sugar patterns on the H molecule into either A, B or both A and B molecules. Possession of the necessary enzymes is inherited in a Mendelian manner (Table 6.1). The determination of the blood group of a patient was normally performed using antibodies obtained from patients who have had incompatible transfusions or who have been immunized specifically for the purpose. Serum samples can be collected, standardized, and used for the testing of red cells by agglutination. Unfortunately such polyclonal antisera have all the disadvantages inherent in non-monoclonal antibodies. There is considerable batch-to-batch variation requiring standardization at each step. The reaction time for agglutination is of the order of 15 min, even with very good antisera. Rapid blood group typing is clearly essential in medical emergencies. Several groups have attempted to make anti-A and anti-B monoclonal antibodies by immunizing animals with cells or purified glycolipids and glycoprotein. One of the products currently being marketed in the U.K. arose accidentally during an experiment designed to look for anti-tumour antibodies. A colorectal tumour cell line, HT29, which grew well in tissue culture, was used to immunize mice in the hope of producing anti-tumour specific antibodies. An antibody was found that bound to tumour cells and also to components in the serum of certain patients, whether or not they had cancer of the colon. Further analysis revealed that the specificity of binding to different cell lines was determined by blood group A. The HT29 cell line was derived from a patient of blood group A. The antibody was found to be a very effective reagent for blood group typing but its properties fell short of polyclonal antisera obtained by hyper-immunizing volunteers. A variety of different immunization schedules were used and anti-A and anti-B monoclonal antibodies are now available which have high affinity and specificity. Not only do the problems of standardization disappear when effective monoclonal antibodies are available, but also the speed of reading the reaction is much greater which is an important factor in emergencies.

Haemolytic disease of the newborn

Another vitally important blood group system was first identified in Rhesus monkeys and is called the rhesus system. Patients are said to be either rhesus negative or rhesus positive depending upon the molecular composition of their red blood cell surface. The rhesus system is important as it is instrumental in inducing haemolytic disease of the newborn. When a rhesus-negative woman is pregnant, with the child of a rhesus-positive man, the fetus may be rhesus positive. Fetal blood cells cross the placenta in small amounts during pregnancy, and in large amounts during labour. A rhesus-negative mother bearing a rhesus-positive child will become immunized to the rhesus antigen. This is of no consequence to the mother or first born child. Subsequent fetuses, however, may develop a severe haemolytic anaemia in utero. The maternal anti-rhesus antibodies which are IgG will freely cross the placenta and haemolyse the red cells of the fetus. The rhesus system is complex and monoclonal antibodies will no doubt allow the further elucidation at a molecular level. Furthermore, there is an opportunity for therapeutic attack. In patients that are rhesus negative it has been shown that the administration of high titre anti-rhesus antibody, prior to the time of maximal transplacental influx of red cells, i.e. prior to labour, will prevent the production of such antibodies by the mother. The immunological mechanism for this is not well understood. It is thought that the high titre antibody administered coats any fetal red cells in the maternal circulation so hiding the rhesus antigens from the mother's immune system. To produce anti-rhesus antibodies, rhesus-negative volunteers (men, who will never become pregnant) are immunized with rhesus-positive red cells. High titre antibodies are produced after several immunizations and serum is collected, purified, and lyophilized ready for use. Again, the polyclonal nature and biological variation of this product makes standardization difficult. Human monoclonal antibodies produced by human hybridomas, obtained by fusing lymphocytes from immunized men, are now available and will soon be used in this clinical situation.

Other blood groups

There are a variety of other glycoprotein and glycolipid antigens such as those of the I, the P, and the MNS system. These antigens may sometimes cause transfusion reactions. Such reactions may be difficult to analyse due to the absence of adequate immunological reagents. Monoclonal antibodies against these will enable the easy typing of blood needed for patients that require multiple transfusions because they have unusual minor blood groups.

Histocompatibility typing

Most of the cells of each individual express antigens which are even more polymorphic than those found on red cells. These antigens were first detected on leucocytes and are called histocompatibility leucocyte antigens (HLA). Although not important during blood transfusion, these antigens are of vital significance during transplantation. Organ transplantation of kidney, liver and bone marrow is becoming an increasingly common procedure, requiring the accurate typing of the HLA expressed on the cells of an individual. Existing serological reagents are obtained by collecting blood from pregnant women who have developed anti-HLA antibodies against paternal HLA types in the fetus and placenta. The nomenclature of the HLA system is confusing, reflecting the complex serological matrices used in its analysis (Fig. 6.4). By making monoclonal antibodies against HLA antigens, a series of standardized reagents are becoming available. Unfortunately, there is a snag. When mice or rats are immunized with HLA molecules, the immune system sees the common determinants in the backbone of the molecule rather than the individual specific determinants. Thus whilst many monoclonal antibodies are available against the backbone of HLA, there are few against the individual determinants. Human monoclonal antibodies may well be required for the dissection of these polymorphic molecules. The use of monoclonal antibodies to distnguish different sub-populations of lymphocytes is considered in Chapter 4.

Lymphocyte differentiation

Over the last 20 years it has become apparent that there are many dif-

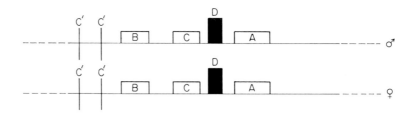

Fig. 6.3. The HLA locus on chromosome 6. There are two alleles, one from each parent. The A, B and C locus products are recognized by antisera. The D locus is analysed by lymphocyte stimulation assays.

ferent types of lymphocyte. These different lymphocytes express patterns of glycoproteins on their cell surface which in turn lead to different functional properties. Investigation of the lymphocyte cell surface has provided important insights into lymphocyte function as well as into the origins of leukaemia and lymphoma. B-lymphocyte sub-populations can be demonstrated by their surface immunoglobulins. Their characterization is made relatively easy by the availability of specific anti-immunoglobulin chain MCA's. Human T-lymphocyte populations have been demonstrated to contain several subsets that differ in function and cell surface characteristics. Unfortunately, the outbred nature of human populations has complicated attempts to develop T-subset-specific antibodies. Prior to the discovery of monoclonal antibodies only limited T-subpopulations could be defined. Now a variety of T-lymphocyte antigens have been defined, present on peripheral blood T-cells at different stages of differentiation (Table 6.2). There are two T-cell antigens present on all T-cells (pan T). Two T-cell subpopulations have also been found that contain lymphocytes with different immuno-regulatory capabilities. A subset bearing a 70,000 dalton glycoprotein, recognized by the OKT8 antibody, has been shown to have killing potential against tumour cells and invading micro-organisms. A second T-cell subset bears a 60,000 molecular weight antigen recognised by the OKT4 antibody. This cell exhibits helper and inducer function. Leukaemias and lymphomas represent the clonal expansion of a single lymphocyte. They therefore express the antigen characteristic of the subset to which the original lymphocyte belonged. The antigenic analysis of lymphocytic malignancy has led to an increase in our understanding of lymphoid

Table 6.2. MCA's recognizing lymphocyte differentiation antigens.

Subset	MCA's
Normal T cells	pan T
T-cell leukaemia	OKT 3
Mycosis fungoides	L17 F12
Helper/inducer T-cells	OKT 4
Sezary syndrome	SK 4
Thymic lymphocytes	OKT 6
Thymoma	
Suppressor/cytotoxic cells	OKT 8
Some T-cell neoplasms	
B lymphocytes and neoplasms	anti-Ig MCA's

differentiation and the origin of different neoplastic types. Using MCA's, leukaemias and lymphomas can be classified providing useful information to the clinician.

MCA's can be used to isolate different subpopulations of lymphocytes using a cell sorter. There are two components to a cell sorter. The first is a flow cytometer which analyses the fluorescence of single cells as they pass through a jet. A suspension of cells mixed with the appropriate fluorescent MCA is injected through a fine nozzle. The kinetics of flow are such that each single microdroplet contains one single cell (Fig. 6.4). As the droplets flow out of the nozzle they are illuminated by an ultraviolet light. A detector picks up the emitted fluorescence. The signals received by the detector are analysed by a computer. A cell will fluoresce when an antibody has bound to its surface. Using electrostatic plates to deflect the droplets, cells can be deviated from their normal pathway when fluorescence occurs. In this way those cells that possess a particular antigen can be separated from those that do not. The cell sorter has proven to be of immense value in understanding the function of different lymphocyte subpopulations. Clearly by separating cells with different surface constituents their function can be analysed at leisure in the laboratory. The technique of cell sorting can be applied to any population of cells whose subcomponents can be identified by suitable

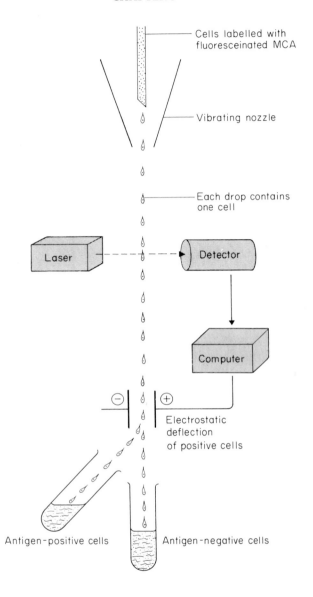

Fig. 6.4. A fluorescence-activated cell sorter. When a cell passes through the laser beam it is monitored for fluorescence. Cells can be deflected depending on the findings of the detector system. All cells possessing a determinant recognized by a fluorescent MCA can thus be isolated.

antibodies. The specificity and homogeneity of monoclonal antibodies make them ideal tools for such an analysis.

Bone marrow transplantation

There are several diseases where the injection of bone marrow from a healthy individual may be of considerable benefit to a patient. These include a wide variety of congenital marrow aplasias where erythrocyte stem cells stop dividing in childhood or adolescence, resulting in severe anaemia. Although such children may be kept alive by frequent blood transfusions, the excess iron in the transfused haemoglobin cannot be excreted. The iron is deposited in liver, muscle and other tissues in the form of haemosiderin. This iron overload eventually leads to functional disorders with serious consequences. These aplasias can be cured if the red cells in the marrow can be replaced by normal stem cells. Disorders of leucocyte and lymphocyte stem cells also occur. These result in impaired defences against invading microorganisms so resulting in severe life-threatening infections. The transfer of stem cells from normal marrow can restore the immune defences. Another use of marrow transplantation is in the treatment of cancer. Current chemotherapy is limited by the tolerance of the stem cells in the marrow which are killed by high doses of cytotoxic drugs. Marrow can be removed from patients and stored prior to aggressive chemotherapy. After this the patients own marrow can be re-infused (cf. Chapter 9).

There are two major problems in marrow transplantation. The first is the rejection of the donor cells by the host. Immunosuppressive therapy is required for a prolonged period of time after transplantation to avoid this. The second problem is more subtle. Transplanted marrow contains T-lymphocytes from the donor. Such cells can recognize the host as foreign, and mount an immune response against host cells. This produces the clinical syndrome of graft-versus-host disease (GVH), with fever, rashes, and liver and kidney failure that may lead to death. Although GVH may be reduced by adequate immunosuppression with newer immunosuppressives such as cyclosporin A, it is still a serious problem in transplantation programmes.

Monoclonal antibodies have three uses in bone marrow transplantation.

1   Accurate tissue typing of **donor** and host lymphocytes. As discussed earlier monoclonal typing reagents are now becoming available which will predict the degree of similarity between HLA of donor and host.

2   Identifying lymphocyte subpopulations in peripheral blood samples. In order to obtain the correct degree of immuno-suppression, varying doses of immuno-suppressive agents such as cyclosporin A and azathioprine are given. By monitoring the levels of different T-lymphocyte subpopulations in the peripheral blood (often expressed as suppressor : cytotoxic cell ratios) information concerning the adequacy of immunosuppression and the likelihood of rejection can be obtained.

3   Removal of T-lymphocytes from donor bone marrow to prevent graft-versus-host disease. Bone marrow removed from a donor is collected and suspended in medium. An anti-T-cell monoclonal antibody is added e.g. OKT3. T-cells can be removed by complement killing, by cell sorting, or by affinity purification on a solid matrix. The T-cell-depleted marrow can then be given to the patient. The incidence of GVH-disease after such pretreatment has been shown to be appreciably less.

Further reading

Anstee D.J (1982) Characterization of human blood groups allo-antigens. In *Monoclonal antibodies in Clinical Medicine*. (Eds A.J. McMichael & J.W. Fabre) p. 237. Academic Press, London.

Festenstein H. & Demant P. (1978) *HLA and H-2*. Edward Arnold, London.

Filipovitch A.H., Ramsay N.K. & Warkentin P.I. (1982) Pretreatment of donor bone marrow with a monoclonal antibody OKT3 for prevention of graft versus host disease. *Lancet* **i**, 1226–1269.

Hoffbrand A.V. & Pettit J.E (1980) *Essential Haematology*. Blackwell Scientific Publications, Oxford.

Schroff R.W., Foon K.A., Billing R.J. & Fahty J.L. (1982) Immunologic classification of lymphocytic leukaemias based on monoclonal-antibody-defined cell surface antigens. *Blood* **56**, 207–215.

Chapter 7

Cell Biology

One of the most remarkable features of a multicellular organism is the difference in structure and function found between cells in different tissues. Differentiation is essential for the continued survival of a large organism, allowing the specialization of function. Nerve, liver and muscle cells, whilst all based on the same general plan, have totally different functions. Differentiation begins during embryogenesis when the stem cells of the fertilized egg start polarizing at one end after reaching the four-cell stage. From then on the switches that are coded for by blocks of genes in the DNA of the cell's nucleus will determine the development of different tissues of an individual.

To the biologist differentiation is a fascinating problem in which the evolution of a species, as well as the individual can be studied. For the clinician, differentiation poses problems in congenital diseases where specific defects occur during embryogenesis, and in cancer where normally differentiated cells start expressing properties associated with earlier stages of development. Modern molecular biology has shown that the reasons for differentiation ultimately reside in the genome. However the end product of gene function is protein. It is the accumulation of different sets of proteins that distinguishes different cells. Each cell possesses the same total DNA content, but the component genes are expressed in varying amounts. The control of gene expression, the conversion of DNA to messenger RNA and hence to protein, is well understood in bacteria. In eukaryotic cells, although the basic steps are understood, the co-ordination of the complex series of switches that occur in producing a muscle or a brain cell remains a mystery (Fig. 7.1). The following three observations, however, are central to the problem of differentiation.

Firstly, a fully differentiated cell can revert under certain circumstances to a less differentiated ancestor. The best example is the insertion of a fully differentiated frog intestinal mucosa cell nucleus into a frog egg whose nucleus has been removed by a micropipette. A normal tadpole will result, indicating that the fully differentiated nucleus possesses all the information required for the production of tissues of all types of differentiation. Although certain gene blocks are

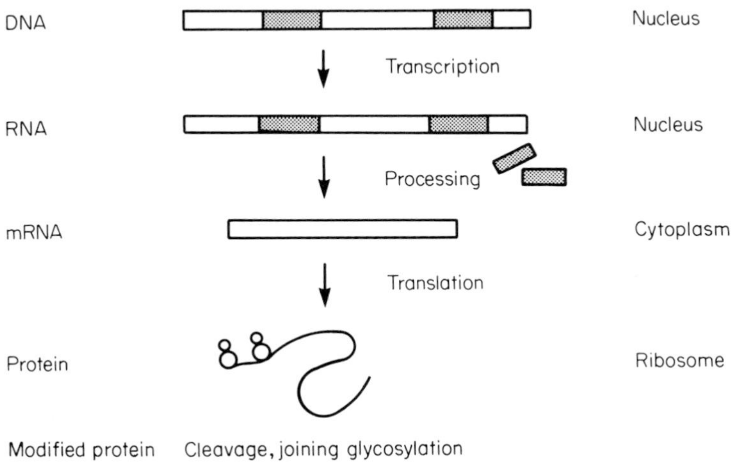

Fig. 7.1. The fundamental steps in protein production from genes in eukaryotes. MCA's are ideal molecular flags for protein.

normally switched on during the process of differentiation, reversion is possible.

A second observation is that the control of gene expression in eukaryotes is at the level of transcription of DNA into messenger RNA (mRNA). The best evidence for this comes from comparing mRNA populations in different tissues using hybridization techniques. Totally different populations are found in liver and brain mRNA, indicating that differentiation results in the production of different sets of mRNA molecules which code for functional proteins. If we could correctly identify these proteins we would understand differentiation.

The third observation is that differentiation results from the planned switching on of gene blocks by gene regulatory proteins in a co-ordinated manner. This is clearly seen in the homeotic mutations of Drosophila, the common fruit fly. Here certain point mutations can cause a leg to be made instead of an antenna giving rise to bizarre insects. This mutation occurs at a single major control site triggering a set of genes that produce limb proteins instead of antenna proteins. This observation illustrates how control of differentiation must occur by combinatorial gene regulation; the interaction of several genes and their products along a defined pathway.

To understand differentiation and its abnormalities we must clearly identify the proteins that characterize different cell types at their various stages of development. Monoclonal antibodies are ideal for this process and are now being used extensively to catalogue the biochemical changes occurring during development. We must define precisely some terms used in cell biology before considering examples of the application of monoclonal antibody technology.

Growth

Growth is defined as the increase in size of an organ or individual, occurring due to an increase in cell size, cell number or by the deposition of synthesized extracellular products in a matrix. The signals that start and stop growth during embryogenesis are not understood but must reside in the ever-changing molecular composition of the cell. Furthermore, once the full adult state is reached growth does not cease. Tissues must be maintained in their differentiated state by the cyclical changes that occur from stem cell turnover to cell death. Repair processes exist to repair damage caused by the external environment.

Hypertrophy

Hypertrophy is the growth of a tissue by the increase in the size of its component cells. An example of this is the increase in muscle bulk in well-trained athletes.

Hyperplasia

Hyperplasia is the growth of tissue by an increase in the number of cells. Hyperplasia occurs cyclically in breast tissue in women in response to hormones released by the ovary. It is also part of the response to tissue damage. An example is the hyperplasia that occurs in the remaining lobe of the liver when one lobe is removed.

Neoplasia

Neoplasia is the uncontrolled growth of cells resulting in a tumour mass. Cancer currently kills one person in five.

Determination

Determination is a self-perpetuating change in the internal character of a cell that distinguishes its progeny from others in the embryo and commits that cell to a particular course of development. The frog nucleus transfer experiment demonstrates that differentiated cells can possess the information required for the full development of a new adult. However, prior to the changes that result in a cell reaching its fully differentiated state, the cells switch on gene blocks that commit them to a particular differentiation pathway, although they are indistinguishable by the cell biologist from their neighbours at that stage.

Differentiation

The specialization of cell character that can be recognized by bio-chemical, morphological, or functional means. The process of differentiation requires the correct genetic switches to be operated in the correct sequence so resulting in the expression of those proteins required to give a differentiated cell its unique character.

Development

Development is the active process of forward change in the life history of an individual from an unicellular zygote to adult life. The term can also be used in an evolutionary sense to follow the development of a species from its ancestors.

Ultimately the control of the protein pattern that makes up an individual cell resides in its DNA. The DNA is transcribed into messenger RNA in the nucleus. After a complex series of processing reactions, similar to the splicing of a film, functional message leaves the pores in the nuclear membrane traversing the endoplasmic reticulum to the ribosomes. These protein factories read the encoded nucleotide sequence in the messenger RNA to produce the amino acid sequence of protein. Proteins that concern us in differentiation are often modified subsequent to their production on the ribosome. This post-translational modification may take the form of cleavage of fragments, the addition of phosphate molecules, or the addition of sugars.

The latter process, called glycosylation, is of fundamental importance.

Glycoproteins

Glycoproteins form the major protein content of the cell surface. It is through the cell surface that a cell interacts with its neighbours and so receives and gives the information concerning differentiation. Recombinant DNA technology provides remarkable tools to study the linear sequence of nucleotides in DNA and RNA and also to characterize the amino acid sequence of proteins. However, the non-linear method by which glycoproteins are synthesized makes their biochemical analysis extremely difficult. The protein moiety is first formed on the ribosome within the endoplasmic reticulum. A standard oligosaccharide is then attached to the asparagine residues of those molecules destined to be glycoproteins (Fig. 7.2). These primitive glycoproteins are transported to the Golgi apparatus in the cell where they are modified. Some of the sugars are removed by glycosylases, whilst other sugars such as glucose, sialic acid and galactose are added by glycosyl transferases. Each glycosyl transferase recognizes, as its specific substrate, the complex of protein with its already attached sugars. The completed molecules are then transported to the surface of the cell where they float on the lipid bilayer membrane. Other important surface determinants include glycolipid. Their biosynthesis is even less well understood. The complex molecular display patterns of the sugar moieties of glycolipids and glycoproteins identifies a cell to the outside world. The analysis of such molecules has been revolutionized by the fine specificity inherent in monoclonal antibody technology as the following examples will show.

Drosophila embryogenesis

The fruitfly, *Drosophila melanogaster*, has been extensively studied by geneticists for more than a century. It breeds rapidly in the laboratory so that large numbers can easily be raised for study. Its genetic map is now well defined and many characterized mutants are available, making it an ideal eukaryote with which to study the translation of genotype into phenotype.

The fundamental problem the cell biologist wishes to address is

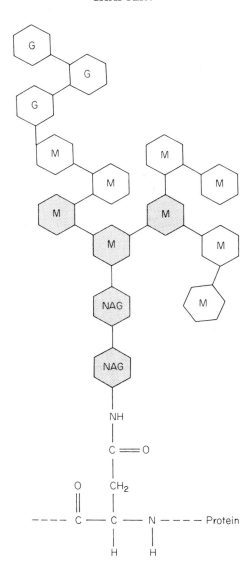

Fig. 7.2. The structure of the asparagine-linked oligosaccharide joined to many proteins in the endoplasmic reticulum. The shaded sugars form the core region which may be built on by glycosyl transferases. The resulting determinants can be identified by MCA's.

how the production of different proteins by normal and mutant genes results in the differences seen in the whole organism. Monoclonal antibodies have now been made against cell surface antigens expressed on embryonic Drosophila cells. To do this, mice were immunized with cells teased out of embryos several hours after fertilization. Antibodies were derived and screened by radioimmunoassay on embryonic cell lines. Immunofluorescence was used to determine the binding pattern of different antibodies on embryos and larval organs. The antigens recognized by the constructed panel of MCA's were found to fall into two categories; those that are ubiquitous on all cells, and those that are limited in their tissue distribution. Tissue-specific antibodies were able to identify molecules that appeared on the cell surface during certain phases of differentiation. Using such techniques, the temporal relationship between the expression of different surface molecules during embryogenesis can now be elucidated.

Teratomas and embryos

One of the first examples of the use of MCA's to explore the expression of different molecules during differentiation came from the same Cambridge laboratory where MCA's were discovered. A set of MCA's was derived by immunizing rats with mouse spleen cells and fusing the immune rat lymphocytes. The original aim of this experiment was to produce reagents to identify mouse lymphocyte subpopulations. The resulting antibodies were also screened for binding on a panel of mouse tumours. One of these antibodies was found to react only with mouse embryonal carcinoma cells and to no other tumour type tested, not even the differentiated derivatives of teratocarcinoma. The molecule which carried the determinant, recognized on embryonal carcinoma cells, was a glycolipid. This appears to be present in stem cell type tumours but not in their differentiated derivatives. The antigen was also found on cells of the pre-implantation mouse embryo. Using indirect immunofluorescence this antigen was first shown to be expressed by all the cells of the early blastocyst stage. The trophectoderm, the precursor of the trophoblast, forms an outer lining to the blastocyst (Fig. 7.3). The antigen detected by the MCA is present on the trophectoderm cells until the blastocyst hatches from the zona pellucida — a protective glycoprotein covering. The inner cell mass

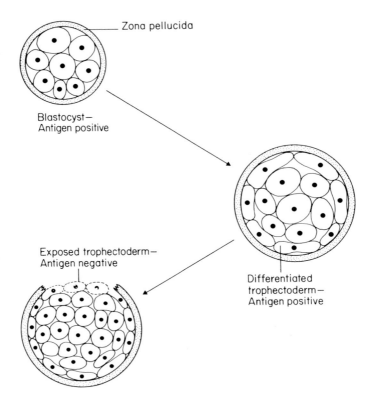

Fig. 7.3. The detection of a phase-specific antigen by a MCA on mouse embryos prior to implantation in the uterus. All cells are positive in the blastocyst stage but lose the antigen when emerging as trophectoderm from the zona pellucida. Such changes are a key to the molecular mechanisms of placental development.

which is destined to become the embryo remains positive at all times. The mechanism by which this antigen disappears is unknown. It appears to be the end product of one of the genetic switches necessary for the development of a functional placenta.

Differentiation in the human brain

The human brain is the most complex biological structure known. Even the simpler nervous systems of lower vertebrates are far more powerful computers than any current man-made machine. Yet the nervous system develops all its connections, both within itself and the end organs, during embryogenesis — a remarkably short time in some species. It is the cell surface that provides the communication mechanism between neurones and glial cells leading to the enactment of the correct 'wiring diagram' for the species. To understand the molecular basis of this process we must identify and characterize the membrane molecules involved in this communication. The monoclonal antibody technology provides an ideal tool for this.

Brain cells and membrane preparations either from whole brain or from specific sites can be used as immunogens. Panels of MCA's can be constructed which will identify subpopulations of cells whose function and development can now be studied. Although such studies are in their infancy, they will almost certainly have a wide ranging impact on neurology.

Further reading

Fabre J.W. (1982) Differentiation antigens of the human central nervous system. In: *Monoclonal Antibodies in Clinical Medicine.* (Eds A.J. McMichael & J.W. Fabre) p. 398–412. Academic Press, London.

Milstein C. & Lennox E. (1980) The use of monoclonal antibody techniques in the study of developing cell surfaces. *Curr. Top. Dev. Biol.* **14**, 1–32.

Neff N.T., Lowrey C., Decker C., Tovar A., Damsky C., Blick C. & Horwitz A.F. (1982) A monoclonal antibody detaches embryonic skeletal muscle from extracellular matrices. *J. Cell. Biol.* **95**, 654–666.

Spragg J.H., Bebbington C.R. & Roberts O.B. (1982) Monoclonal antibodies recognizing cell surface antigens in Drosophila melanogaster. *Develop. Biol.* **89**, 339–352.

Willison K.R. & Stern P.L. (1978) Expression of Forsmann antigenic specificity in the preimplantation mouse embryo. *Cell,* **14**, 785–793.

Chapter 8

Cancer Localization

Cancer is caused by the abnormal proliferation of cells. There are two types of tumour. The first is benign. Although such tumours may grow fairly rapidly, they remain localized to their site of origin and do not invade adjacent organs. Their symptoms are caused by local pressure and treatment is by surgical removal. Complete recovery of the patient is the rule. Malignant tumours, on the other hand, are characterized by their ability to grow rapidly, to invade adjacent organs and tissues, and to spread throughout the blood or lymphatic system to establish distant colonies of tumour known as metastases. It is the presence or absence of these metastases which often determines whether patients suffering from malignant tumours will live or die. Such metastases may in themselves give rise to further spread of tumour. Although the primary tumour may be eradicated by surgery or radiotherapy, the metastases will remain unaffected. It is the metastatic tumour that ultimately causes treatment failure and kills the patient.

To the clinician treating patients with malignant tumours it is clearly of great importance to establish whether or not an individual patient has metastatic disease. This is true, both at the time of diagnosis when treatment is being planned, and also afterwards when the patient is being regularly reviewed by his physician. Many investigations are currently available to help in the follow up of cancer patients. These include the measurement of enzymes and protein products in the blood, which will determine liver and kidney function; and conventional X-rays and computerized tomography scans (CT), which are capable of detecting areas of abnormality greater than at least 0.5 cm in diameter. Similarly, nuclear medicine has contributed greatly to the management of patients with malignant disease by the development of techniques such as isotope bone and liver scanning. Here a radioactive material which is taken up by the organ is given and areas of abnormality due to the presence of tumour will show up either as increased or decreased uptake on a scan of radioactivity distribution in the patients. These scans detect areas of abnormality with great precision and reproducibility. The limitation with all these methods is that the abnormalities detected are non-specific. Similar

X-ray or scan appearances may be produced by tumours, abscesses, cysts and certain congenital malformations. What is required in clinical practice is the development of techniques which specifically detect tumours and will reliably and safely allow the physician to discover if his patient has evidence of active malignant disease. Such specific substances are usually called tumour markers and, in many cases, their place in clinical medicine is already well established. An example is carcinoembryonic antigen (CEA) in colon cancer. CEA is shed by the cancer cells into the blood and a rise in its level in a blood sample heralds the recurrence of malignant disease in a particular patient (Chapter 3). The detection of such circulating tumour markers has been greatly facilitated by the development of specific MCA's. In this chapter we review the use of MCA's to tumour-associated antigens to locate malignant cells within patients suffering from certain types of cancer.

Antibodies to cancer cells

There is considerable evidence that the immune system is able to recognize tumours as being different from normal tissue. However, the strength of the signal to the immune system from most tumours, both in humans and laboratory animals, appears to be very weak. There is little evidence that the immune defence mechanisms are able to successfully inhibit neoplastic growth once a tumour has developed. The ability of a malignant cell to stimulate a host response must arise from differences between the molecular composition of the cell surface compared to that of its normal counterpart. Throughout this century many attempts have been made to stimulate the body's immune reaction to cancer cells to destroy metastases. However, little impact on treatment has been made. Part of the problem is the complexity of the immune system. The monoclonal antibody technology now offers hope that such complex systems may be broken down into their constituent parts and used to help treat patients with malignant disease. In this way we may be able to analyse the very small differences between tumour and normal cells. There are now many reports of MCA's being raised against human solid and blood malignancies.

Tumour-associated antigens

All clinical work utilizing MCA's to recognize tumours is based on the assumption that antigens exist on the malignant cell which are not present on its normal counterpart. It is accepted that such differences may be very subtle indeed. Much of the investigative work has been directed towards the detection of tumour-specific antigens, i.e. antigens which are present and expressed only when malignant transformation has occurred in a cell and are never found in the normal cell. So far there is no real evidence that any such tumour-specific antigen exists in human cancer although the search continues (Table 8.1). Most work has been concerned with tumour-associated antigens, i.e. antigens which are expressed in minute quantities in the normal cell but are expressed in much greater quantity when malignant transformation has taken place. Such changes may reflect secondary characteristics of the malignant cell, such as degree of differentiation or rate of division. None the less, several of these tumour-associated antigens have been described in certain tumours and can be used for diagnostic techniques. An example is alpha-fetoprotein which is normally only detected during fetal life and in the developing liver. Its presence on hepatomas and teratomas may be explained by the increased degree of cell turnover which occurs in both embryos and tumours.

Antibody production

Before embarking upon the production of a monoclonal antibody for clinical work it is necessary to consider for what purpose such an antibody is required. Antibodies which appear to have ideal properties in laboratory testing for binding to tumours may well behave differently when administered to patients. It is obvious that different properties will be required from an antibody, which is to be used for clinical

Table 8.1. Surface antigens on cancer cells

Histocompatibility antigens
Tumour-specific transplantation antigens
Embryonic antigens
Viral antigens
Differentiation antigens

tumour localization, than from an antibody which is to be used as a stain to detect the presence of tumour cells in a tissue biopsy. The perfect antibody for tumour localization would be totally tumour specific with a high binding affinity to an antigen present in great quantity on all tumour cells but on no normal tissues. It should be an IgG antibody because the relatively low molecular weight of this antibody subclass would allow free diffusion within the body. It should also be secreted in high concentration by a stable hybridoma line so that production problems are minimized. The line should be capable of growth in serum-free medium to enable its complete purification. In this way no impurities would be given to patients with their attendant side-effects.

Scanning technique

If an antibody can be prepared which is capable of recognizing tumour cells, but has little or no cross-reaction to any normal human tissue, it may be suitable for scanning. In principle a radioactive isotope may be attached to a monoclonal antibody in such a fashion that the immuno-reactivity of the antibody, as defined by in vitro binding assays, is unaltered. If such a labelled antibody is then injected into the patient, after a suitable time the antibody will bind to tumour-associated antigens in the patient. The localization of this antibody–antigen complex can be detected by an external radiation camera and an image produced of the patient's body outline with the position of the labelled antibody–antigen complexes. It is correct to think of such scans as antigen distribution images where the molecule being imaged is in fact the tumour-associated antigen. However, under physiological circumstances this antigen is present not only on the tumour itself. As tumour cells die and are replaced some antigen is shed into the patient's blood stream and may circulate in relatively large concentration around the patient's body (the presence of such circulating antigen forms the basis for the detection of tumour markers). Therefore the scan obtained will reflect the distribution of the antigen both on the tumour and in the blood stream. In order to turn this into a clinically useful image the technique of subtraction scanning is necessary. In this, a second isotope is injected into the patient 48 hr after the injection of the labelled monoclonal antibody. This second isotope is of a significantly different energy from the first isotope and is attached to a carrier which is designed to stay within the circulating blood pool of the patient. The images of both isotopes are recorded simultaneously on two separate channels of a suitable radiation detector, such as a rectilinear scanner. The first and higher-energy-labelled monoclonal antibody will demonstrate the presence of tumour plus blood pool, whilst the second, lower energy isotope should delineate the presence of blood pool alone. Using standard nuclear medicine computer programmes it is possible to subtract the second image from the first, thus leaving an image of the tumour alone (Plate 2). Although such subtraction techniques are widely practised in hospital nuclear medicine departments, they require complex and expensive equipment and as such limit the performance of isotope scans to centres which possess this equipment.

Scanning colorectal cancer

As an example of the development and use of monoclonal antibodies for scanning we describe our experience in colorectal cancer. Antibodies for scanning were prepared by immunizing rats with solubilized membrane preparations from a fresh specimen of a human colorectal carcinoma. After hybridization of the rat splenic lymphocytes with a rat myeloma line, hybrid cells were selected for cloning on the basis of *in vitro* binding in a radioimmunoassay to HT29 cells, a human colorectal cell line. A panel of nine antibodies were chosen which appeared to recognize colorectal tumour cells and had very little activity against normal colon tissue. Screening to select the

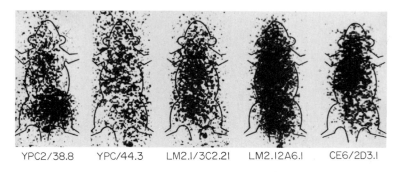

YPC2/38.8   YPC/44.3   LM2.I/3C2.2I   LM2.I2A6.I   CE6/2D3.I

Fig. 8.1. Mice bearing human colorectal tumour xenografts injected with various radiolabelled MCA's. YPC2/38.8 shows good localization of tumour.

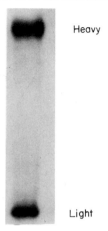

Fig. 8.2. Radiolabelled MCA obtained by labelling purified Ig from hybridoma cells growing in serum-free medium. Autoradiography of SDS-polyacrylamide gel electrophoresis shows two bands corresponding to heavy and light chains of Ig.

best antibody was performed *in vitro* by means of immunofluorescence and immunoperoxidase staining and also by radioimmunoassay (cf. Chapter 4). *In vivo* recognition of colorectal tumours was tested by scanning immuno-deficient mice bearing human colon tumours as xenografts. These mice were injected 48 hr previously with the labelled monoclonal antibody (Fig. 8.1). From this, one antibody (YPC2/12.1.) was chosen for further work in patients. For implementation of the subtraction technique, outlined above, the antibody was labelled with [131]Iodine (energy 330KV) at a specific activity of 1 mCi ^{131}I/mg immunoglobulin (Fig. 8.2). Patients with known advanced colorectal cancer were injected with this antibody. None experienced any unpleasant side-effects or symptoms. For background subtraction of the blood pool the patients received an injection of 0.5 mCi of [99M]Technetium pertechnetate and 0.5 mCi of [99M]Technetium-labelled human serum albumen. Prior to any isotope injection the patients were given potassium iodide tablets in order to block thyroid uptake of any free iodine in the injected material. Forty-eight hours after injection of the labelled isotope, patients were scanned using a rectilinear scanner and data recorded on a computer looking at the iodine and technetium channels simultaneously. Using the background subtraction method, images were then produced by a

91

colour printer to determine areas of relatively high differential activity. Using this method, areas of tumour were successfully identified in most patients. An example is shown in Plate 3. Reasons for failure in some patients include the administration of prior radiotherapy to the site of the lesion which clearly affects the distribution of the tumour-associated antigens and thus the image.

Problems with scanning

Problems related to radiolabelled monoclonal antibodies can be divided into those concerning the antibody itself and those concerned with the techniques used to image tumours. Firstly, antibodies used in all series so far are only operationally tumour specific. This means that they will recognize tumours better than normal tissue but their activity is not exclusively directed against the tumour. Some of the distribution of the antibody within the patient must represent non-specific binding of the immunoglobulin by its Fc terminal. Therefore the preparation of $(Fab)_2$ fragments (cf. Chapter 1) of the same immunoglobulin may eliminate much of the this non-specific binding activity. For similar reasons it may be better to use, as the subtraction agent, a Technetium-labelled irrelevant monoclonal antibody of the same subclass. However, for chemical reasons it has so far proved impossible to produce stable Technetium immunoglobulin conjugates and therefore this technique has not yet found a place in routine clinical practice. There is also the worry about a host reaction to a foreign rat or mouse protein. Because of this many clinical investigators have found it necessary to administer labelled antibodies slowly with intravenous infusions covered by steroid and antihistamine preparations. This precaution adds considerably to the complexity of a routine clinical investigation.

As far as the methodology of tumour localization is concerned the need for some subtraction techniques is unsatisfactory. This is because the technique relies upon the use of two isotopes whose energies must be sufficiently different for the computer to be able to recognize areas of differential activity. In the case ^{131}Iodine and ^{99M}Technetium the more energetic iodine scatters outside the patient's body whereas the less energetic ^{99M}Technetium will not scatter so far and therefore the computer will show areas of differential activity which are outside the patient's body; the halo effect. Although this is easy to ignore with practice, it is a source of confusion to many clinicians when first presented with monoclonal antibody scans. Similarly, as the subtraction technique demonstrates areas of differential activity between the two agents, it is possible to produce an image by virtue of the absence of Technetium in an area deprived of blood supply. Although such areas are rare within the body, the possibility of negative Technetium activity must be considered when viewing all areas of apparent labelled antibody uptake on the final subtraction scan.

For all these reasons it would be more satisfactory to develop methods which could be independent of subtraction techniques. At present the most promising method involves the use of emission tomography scanning. By this method, transverse 'slices' of the body can be examined by a gamma camera which is rotating around the central long-axis of the patient. This method allows for greater resolution of small areas of uptake and is capable of distinguishing between activity of the labelled antibody in tumour and blood by viewing suspicious areas from all angles.

The most satisfactory way to produce better scans would be by the development of antibodies which were truly capable of recognizing tumour cells and not normal tissue. In addition these antibodies should bind with great affinity to the tumour cell and be rapidly excreted from the blood when circulating in a free state. The hope that such antibodies may already exist against certain tumour types is becoming stronger. More recently there have been exciting reports that human monoclonal antibodies raised against certain types of brain tumours, called gliomas, have shown selective concentration within the tumour itself with little or no activity in the cerebrospinal fluid or peripheral blood. Human monoclonal antibodies would also have the advantage that, as human proteins they would not be likely to stimulate a foreign protein reaction in the host and hypersensitivity would be avoided. The use of human monoclonal antibodies for tumour localization is discussed in Chapter 10.

Conclusion

Labelled monoclonal antibody scanning gives the clinician a powerful tool for the recognition and localization of malignant cells within a patient's body. Although certain technical problems still exist, the next few years should see a rapid expansion of experimental work in this area. This technique could become a routine investigation in the management of patients with malignant disease. The use of labelled antibodies to study the distribution and activity of antigens under different physiological conditions in patients could provide interesting results in areas other than cancer. Furthermore the same monoclonal antibodies can carry not only diagnostic isotopes but therapeutic agents such as drugs, toxins or high activity radioisotopes. In this way monoclonal antibodies could be used to target therapy specifically onto tumour cells, thus providing the clinician with a therapeutic weapon more specific than anything available today.

Further reading

Berche C., Mach J.P., Lumbroso J.D., Langlais C., Aubry L., Carrel S. & Parmentier C. (1982) Tomoscintigraphs for detecting gastrointestinal and medullary thyroid cancers. *Brit. Med. J.* **285**, 1447–1451.

Deland F.H., Kim E., Simmons G. & Goldenberg D.M. (1980) Imaging approach in radioimmunodetection. *Cancer Res.* **40**, 3046–3049.

Larson S.M. (1983) Imaging of malanoma with ^{131}I-labelled monoclonal antibodies. *J. Nucl. Med.* **24**, 123–129.

Mach, J.P., Finan P., Lennox E.S., Ritson A., Sikora K. & Wraight P. (1981) Use of radiolabelled monoclonal anti-CEA antibodies for the detection of human carcinomas by external photoscanning and tomoscintigraphy. *Immunol. Today*, **2**, 239–249.

Smedley, H.M. *et al.* (1983) Localisation of colorectal carcinoma by a radiolabelled monoclonal antibody. *Brit. J. Cancer*, **47**, 253–260.

Chapter 9

Cancer Treatment

The clinical practice of administering chemicals to patients for the treatment of disease is known as chemotherapy and the academic study of such chemicals as pharmacology. A major problem is the specificity of the drugs employed. It is now clear from extensive clinical experience that any chemical introduced into a patient will have a multiplicity of actions. Some may be desirable and some undesirable. It is the balance between these two effects which determines whether or not a particular drug is considered clinically useful. If morphine is given to a patient in order to relieve severe pain, then its other effect of causing constipation may be regarded as a side-effect. However, the same action may be usefully employed when treating a patient with diarrhoea, when its action in causing constipation is advantageous. Under ideal circumstances we would like to administer drugs which exert only one single effect on the body and that this would be adequate to treat the particular symptom or disease from which the patient was suffering. However, no such drugs exist for cancer.

Problems in cancer treatment

A major problem in treating patients with cancer is our inability to selectively destroy metastatic neoplastic cells. Surgery and radiotherapy are often effective in eradicating primary tumours. Increased awareness of cancer over the last two decades, both amongst the public and physicians, has resulted in the presentation of malignant disease at an earlier stage. Despite this, nearly 50% of patients with common solid tumours have metastatic disease at the time of presentation. Screening programmes and increased public awareness are unlikely to change this statistic significantly. Variations in the way in which physicians deal with the primary disease can have no effect on the survival of patients with metastases. This is exemplified in breast cancer where considerable controversy has been generated about the best way to use combinations of surgery and radiotherapy. The end results, however, remain constant with 40% of patients dying within 5 years. The treatment of metastatic disease clearly requires systemic therapy. For this to be effective it must discriminate between malignant and non-malignant cells. Chemo- and endocrine therapy can often do this, but unfortunately neoplastic cells can rapidly devise mechanisms to resist therapy. Most chemotherapeutic regimes are empirical, with drug combinations designed to avoid additive toxicity.

The current treatment of metastatic disease for common solid tumours can be compared to the treatment of infectious diseases in the pre-antibiotic era of the 1930s. The differences between behaviour of the malignant cell and its normal counterpart are so subtle that any drug which is capable of destroying malignant cells, will undoubtedly also have a significant effect on a large number of normal cells. This unwanted toxicity on the normal cells may require the cancer treatment to be stopped. For example an ovarian carcinoma may be treated by chlorambucil which is taken daily by mouth. Chlorambucil is effective in destroying proliferating cells but is particularly active against cells of the lymphoid series when given in doses large enough to be effective against the ovarian tumour. It may also cause a significant depression of the circulating white cell count and thus render the patient liable to infection and death due to septicaemia. Such toxicities are limiting in employing drugs against certain malignant diseases. All drugs effective against cancer have considerable side-effects on normal tissue which may in themselves be extremely hazardous for the patient. It is for this reason that their use is restricted to physicians who are specially trained and experienced. One example of a dose-limiting toxicity is adriamycin, an antibiotic active against breast cancer. This causes complete hair loss and damage to the muscles of the heart. Another is in *cis*-dichlorodiaminoplatinum, a compound extremely valuable in the treatment of malignant teratomas, which causes renal damage. It is therefore not surprising that considerable energy and research is spent in trying to produce drugs which are more specific in their action and which would have less toxicity. So far this effort has gone largely unrewarded. The use of MCA's may represent an alternative strategy whereby the selective action of drugs may be increased for therapeutic benefit. Table 9.1 summarizes the potential of MCA's in clinical oncology.

Let us consider the use of adriamycin in the treatment of breast

Table 9.1. Potential uses of monoclonal antibodies in oncology

Areas of potential use	Specific use
Diagnosis	
Circulating tumour markers	Screening
	Diagnosis
	Monitoring
	Prognosis
	Treatment decisions
Histology	Prognosis
	Treatment Decisions
Cytology	Sputum
	Urine
	Vaginal smears,
	Effusions and bone marrow
Immunoscintigraphy	Detection
	Localization
Therapy	
Bone marrow clearance	
Systemic Therapy	Antibody alone
	Coupled
	Drugs
	Toxins
	Radionucleides

cancer. The drug belongs to a group of anti-cancer agents known as anthracycline antibiotics, and was originally isolated from a mutant strain of Streptomyces peucetius in the mid-1960s. Adriamycin has shown itself to be one of the most consistently effective drugs in the treatment of solid tumours when used alone or in combination with other drugs. However, it is associated with certain hazards immediately after administration to patients. They feel nauseated and frequently vomit, and develop complete loss of hair. This symptom alone can be psychologically very distressing for a patient already suffering from malignant disease. More importantly it has been shown to have a specific action on the muscle of the heart (myocardium) and for this reason it is ncessary to constantly monitor the patients with electrocardiograms during adriamycin treatment and to limit the total dose to around 1000 mg in any individual patient. Beyond this dose, acute heart failure and sudden death may occur. These distressing effects combine to limit the dose that can be given. When used alone in breast cancer, objective regression occurs in 40% of patients and it is not unreasonable to hope that if the dose and frequency of this drug delivered to the tumour could be increased then this response rate may also be improved. If an antibody were raised which could recognize breast tissue, then such an antibody when injected into a patient would localize to the tumour and/or normal breast tissue. If, prior to the injection of a breast-seeking antibody, adriamycin were to be conjugated chemically to the antibody in such a way that the antibody retained all its immunoreactivity, then it is possible that the antibody could act as a vehicle for targeting the drug onto the required tissue. This may have the effect of producing a high concentration of active drug within breast tissue while leaving little or no drug present in the general systemic circulation.

The advantages of such a delivery system can instantly be seen. Firstly it may be possible to produce, within the tumour, higher concentrations of active drug than are possible at present by intravenous injection, thus making the efficacy of the drug greater. Secondly, by reducing the circulating adriamycin to minute levels, much of the toxicity presently encountered may be avoided. This would make the drug safer to give, as well as being more acceptable to the patient. Methods for conjugating drugs onto antibodies have also been developed with considerable success. One remaining difficulty, however, is the uncoupling of the drug from the antibody when it reaches the target site. This step is necessary because most anti-tumour antibodies are directed against cell surface antigens. On the other hand, most anti-cancer drugs such as adriamycin need to gain entry into the cell itself. Therefore a major hurdle is to devise a method by which the active drug will become disassociated from its carrier antibody when the latter reaches its target on the cancer cell surface.

Production of the antibody

It should be noted in the above example that reference is made to a tissue-associated antigen rather than a tumour-associated antigen. This is because many tumours arise from normal tissues and organs whose function is crucial to the survival of the individual, e.g. brain or liver, and therefore when we talk about tumour-associated antigens we are seeking to exploit an immunological difference between a tumour cell and its normal counterpart. Only in this way is it possible to direct therapy against the malignant cell whilst hoping to leave normal healthy tissue intact and functioning. However, in the case of breast cancer this distinction is not necessary as normal breast tissue is not essential for the survival of the individual. It would be perfectly satisfactory at an operational level to produce an antibody which was capable of distinguishing breast tissue from all other normal tissues. It would be of no consequence to the individual if such an antibody was used to target an agent which caused destruction not only of the malignant breast tissue but also of all normal breast tissue as well. This significant biological advantage has already been successfully used to produce antibodies capable of recognizing breast tissue by immunizing with cell products such as milk fat globulin. Antibodies made in this way can be used in the diagnosis and staging of patients with breast cancer. As discussed in Chapter 1 it is important to define what function is required of an antibody prior to its use in any given clinical situation.

Tumour-specific antibodies

Tumours arise in tissues that are vital to survival such as the lung, colon and blood cells. Clearly in these diseases a truly tumour-specific antibody must be constructed. The molecular composition of the tumour cell surface differs from that of its normal counterpart. These differences can be detected by the effector arms of the immune response, both humoral and cellular. Although there is considerable evidence that the immune system can recognize the tumour cell surface as abnormal, there is little evidence that once a tumour has developed, effector mechanisms are able to inhibit successfully neo-plastic growth. Over the last century many investigators have tried to augment the specific response of the immune system, to provide selective tumour destruction in both animal systems and patients with cancer. A major problem has been the complexity of the immune system and our inability to break it down into its individual components. Antibodies raised in a variety of animal species have been used in attempts to treat patients with cancer with little success. These sera have been prepared by immunizing animals with human tumour material and then absorbing the sera with normal human tissue to remove anti-human activity and, it was hoped, to leave behind specific anti-tumour activity. In most cases, however, such absorption removes most of the activity and therefore such sera are unlikely to be effective. The monoclonal antibody technology yields unlimited quantities of pure reagents which avoid crossreaction from contaminating antibodies and offers the best hope of providing reagents that will selectively recognize tumour cell surfaces. There have been many reports on the production of monoclonal antibodies to human solid tumours.

Before describing laboratory strategies for producing and selecting suitable MCA's, it is useful to consider the attributes of a perfect MCA for use in clinical oncology. Human MCA's have the attraction of not eliciting an immune response when administered to patients, with resulting abrogation of their effects and the problems of unpleasant immune complex phenomena. A perfect MCA should clearly be totally tumour specific with a high binding affinity to an antigen present in abundance on all tumour cells and no normal tissue. An IgG antibody has advantages compared with an IgM, as its relatively low molecular weight will allow free diffusion within the extracellular space. The MCA should be secreted in high concentration by a hybridoma line which should grow in serum-free medium to enable complete purification of secreted antibody.

Immunization schedules for preparing MCA's to human tumour surface antigens have varied widely. Very little detailed work has been performed on optimizing the schedules. Different groups have used different sources of tumour material, whole cells, membranes or solubilised products, either derived from cell lines or from clinical biopsy samples (Fig. 9.1). Mice and rats have been immunized, using different timing schedules and different routes of immunization which will almost certainly produce different spectra of antibodies. In preparing human hybridomas no immunization is possible but there is a choice in the source of lymphocytes used for fusion.

Techniques have been developed to enhance the frequency of antigen-specific hybridomas. One is to enrich for antibody-producing lymphocytes prior to cell fusion. Spleen cells from animals immunized with haptens such as dinitrophenol can be cultured in vitro for 4 days in the presence of the immunizing antigen or transferred into x-irradiated syngeneic recipients, followed by an in vivo antigen boost 4 days prior to their use in cell fusion. Both procedures decrease the total number of cells available for hybridization, but increase the percentage of antigen-specific, antibody-secreting clones following

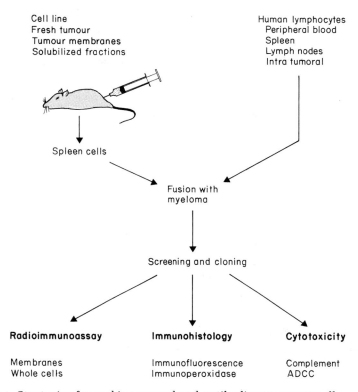

Fig. 9.1. Strategies for making monoclonal antibodies to cancer cells.

cell fusion. Such techniques are now being investigated for the production of anti-tumour MCA's.

Screening

Whichever immunization schedule and fusion system are used, the eventual spectrum of MCA's produced against any antigen will depend upon the methods used for screening to find suitable immunoglobulins. There are three main screening methods: radioimmunoassay by binding to membranes or whole cell lines; immunohistology using either fluorescence or peroxidase techniques; and cytotoxicity either by the addition of complement or by antibody-dependent cellmediated cytotoxicity. In searching for anti-human tumour MCA's,

101

there are advantages in the use of immunohistology in a primary screen (cf. Chapter 4). As well as providing a rapid screening technique, this method also allows the acquisition of information about the exact location of an antigen and its distribution within a tumour. Binding radioimmunoassasys provide the most rapid way of screening large numbers of supernatants for antibody activity, but may not pick up all antibodies that have clinical use, such as those which activate cell-mediated cytotoxicity.

Specificity

Although it is relatively easy to construct sets of MCA's which have activity against a particular tumour, it is much more difficult to characterize specificity and produce antibodies reacting with defined target antigens. The most common method to characterize MCA's is to study binding to a panel of different cell lines. Unfortunately by increasing the sensitivity of these binding assays, apparent specificity often disappears.

The search for MCA's with well defined specificity is clearly essential if antibodies are to be of use for targeting drugs or toxic agents. For tumour localization, or in vitro removal of tumour cells from bone marrow during autologous marrow transplantation, fine specificity may not be so essential for clinical usefulness.

Destruction of malignant cells in bone marrow

Bone marrow provides a repository for tumour cells from a variety of malignancies. Bone marrow can be relatively easily collected and stored from a patient, whilst aggressive radiotherapy and chemo-therapy can be administered at a dose which would normally be lethal to the patient because of marrow toxicity. Following such therapy, the patient can be given back his own marrow. The problem at present with this technique, which has now been attempted in leukaemias and also some solid tumours, is that the re-infused marrow may contain tumour cells. In vitro treatment of a marrow suspension with a monoclonal antibody may remove these cells. There are two problems with this approach; the first is that even the most aggressive radiotherapy and chemotherapy may not effectively destroy all tumour cells present in the body. The total dose of drugs and radiation is still limited by other rapid turn-over organ systems, such as the gut and skin epithelium. The second problem is ensuring that every single tumour cell is removed from the marrow before re-infusion. Although it is relatively easy to separate a few tumour cells from 10^7 marrow cells, scaling up to handle 10^{10} cells poses considerable technical difficulties. Clinical trials using this approach are now under way in breast and lung cancer.

Systemic therapy with monoclonal antibodies

Lymphoma

The first published clinical study on the therapeutic use of a MCA was in a patient with non-Hodgkin's lymphoma. These lymphomas are a mixed group of diseases in which neoplastic lymphocytes develop, usually in lymph nodes, but subsequently spread to other organs including the blood and marrow. The first patient was a 54-year-old man with a 1-year history of lymph node enlargement with liver and spleen involvement. After extensive chemotherapy with many different drugs the patient developed an unresponsive lymphoma-cell leukaemia. A mouse MCA against tumour cells from this patient, had been derived a year previously, which bound to a limited subset of B-cell non-Hodgkin's lymphomas. A total of 250 mg of purified antibody was given by intravenous infusion to the patient with no untoward side-effects over a 60-hr period. Tumour cells were transiently cleared from the circulation but antibody activity was abrogated by a circulating blocking antigen, presumably shed by tumour cell membranes. Following this study, a total dose of 2 g of the antibody was administered in two courses in the subsequent 3 weeks, again without significant toxicity. Although there was some transient change in the condition of the patient, the tumour eventually grew out of control and the patient died. Factors contributing to the failure of therapy probably included the large number of tumour cells present, the weak expression on the cell surface of the tumour antigen and the quantity of circulating antigen which blocked tumour cell binding. The mechanism of cell destruction was almost certainly complement-mediated cytotoxicity.

T-cell leukaemia

Another murine monoclonal antibody which reacts with a normal human T-cell differentiation antigen was used to treat patients with Sézary syndrome. This rare condition is a lymphoma-cell leukaemia that occurs in about 5% of patients with the T-helper cell lymphoma, mycosis fungoides. Initially this disease effects the skin, with widespread infiltration in the epidermis. As the disease progresses it may involve lymph nodes, viscera, and bone marrow. The patient's circulating lymphoma cells were shown to contain large amounts of antigen recognized by the antibody using immunofluorescence. Prior to therapy, circulating antigen was not detectable in the serum using a competition radioimmunoassay. After two courses of intravenous therapy with a total of 7 mg of antibody, there was a dramatic fall in the abnormal circulating cell count but this returned to pre-treatment levels within 48 hr. After the first dose of antibody, circulating free antigen and a transient impairment in renal function were noted. The latter suggested immune complex formation. At various times during and after antibody therapy the patient's cells were incubated with the antibody and studied by quantitative immunofluorescence using flow cytometry. Loss of the antigen by leukaemia cells (antigenic modulation) was found transiently following each course of therapy. Other patients with florid skin manifestations of mycosis fungoides were treated. Transient clinical and histological regressions were noted after antibody therapy.

Acute lymphoblastic leukaemia

Several patients with acute lymphoblastic leukaemia, both children and adults, have been given a MCA specific for the common acute lymphoblastic leukaemia antigen, CALLA. There was a rapid decrease in circulating blast cells in several patients that began immediately after antibody infusion. Not all the leukaemia cells were cleared and the remaining cells appeared to be resistant to further therapy.

Chronic lymphoblastic leukaemia

Several patients with chronic lymphocytic leukaemia (CLL), again extensively treated with chemotherapy, had been given i.v. infusions of a murine MCA to an antigen on the surface of CLL cells, normal and malignant T-cells and thymocytes. There was a marked fall in the abnormal circulating cells with a prompt return within several hours to the previously raised level. A serious anaphylactic reaction developed in one patient on the third infusion of 10 mg of MCA, with urticaria, diarrhoea, dyspnoea and a fall in blood pressure. This responded rapidly to adrenalin, corticosteroids and plasma volume expansion. In vivo binding of antibody was demonstrated with subsequent tumour cell lysis.

Colorectal carcinoma

There are very few studies of monoclonal antibody therapy in patients with common solid tumours. A series of MCA's binding to human colorectal carcinoma have been studied. One of these antibodies has been shown to activate antibody-dependent cell-mediated cytotoxicity by both mouse and human effector cells. The administration of this antibody to mice, bearing human colorectal carcinoma xenografts, inhibited tumour growth. Furthermore, this antibody perfused through freshly resected human colons containing adenocarcinomas selectively bound to cells of some of these tumours. A clinical trial of this antibody in the treatment of gastrointestinal tumours has been performed in four patients who were given 15–200 mg of purified antibody. There was very little objective evidence of tumour regression. In one patient, who received autologous mononuclear cells that had been mixed with the monoclonal antibody into a hepatic artery catheter, the hepatic metastases became smaller and there was a change in the pattern of infiltrating host cells of a resected metastasis.

Malignant melanoma

An evaluation to assess the toxicity and kinetics of a MCA specific for a melanoma-associated antigen was carried out in two patients with end-stage melanoma. Both patients had extensive disease and had failed to respond to all conventional chemotherapy. The patients received 10 mg doses of the antibody intravenously over a 2-hr period. Subcutaneous tumour biopsies failed to show evidence of in vivo tumour binding. No major toxicity was observed. There was no evidence of tumour cell destruction.

Arming monoclonal antibodies

Over the next few years it is likely that different monoclonal antibodies will find a routine place in the diagnosis and evaluation of cancer patients. Whether they will also have a role in delivering effective systemic therapy for metastatic disease remains to be seen. There are several mechanisms by which the administration of a suitable monoclonal antibody can result in tumour cell death, most of which are discussed in detail elsewhere in this volume. Unfortunately, there are also mechanisms by which tumour cells can overcome this attack (Table 9.2). Cells can evolve out of the unfavourable influence of a destructive antibody by changing the composition of their surface. To ensure rapid killing, drugs, toxins and radionucleides can be coupled to MCA's in such a way that their immunological activity remains unaltered. The antibody therefore provides a targeting mechanism whilst the coupled agent acts as a warhead.

Physical agents

Once the principle of targeting therapy to a required area of disease, in order to increase the specificity of action of therapeutic agents, is established, it is clear that several types of agent can be used. Great interest has been shown in the use of radioactive isotopes. Let us first

Table 9.2. Problems in MCA therapy for cancer

1.	Immune complex formation of MCA
2.	Poor vascularity of tumour
3.	Patchy antigen distribution in tumour
4.	Internalization of antigen on exposure to MCA
5.	Antigen shedding by tumour — 'smokescreen effect'
6.	Evolution of antigen negative clones

consider the ideal properties required of a radioactive isotope prior to its administration for targeted cancer therapy.

Some elements have inherently unstable proton and neutron combinations and may change their own atomic structure to achieve a more stable combination. During such changes atoms emit energy which is capable of penetrating solid material; a phenomena known as radioactivity. Three main types of radioactive emissions are recognized.

1   Alpha particle: This is a positively charged particle with a mass identical to a helium nucleus. This is the largest and heaviest of all the radioactive particles encountered and although it is capable of only very limited penetration, it will do great damage to any cell which it enters. It has a high *linear energy transfer* (i.e. it deposits considerable energy along its path).

2   Beta particle: A beta particle is an electron — a negatively charged particle with virtually no mass. Although the energy of electrons is high, their small mass results in low *linear energy transfer* and therefore they cause less biological damage than alpha particles.

3   Gamma rays: Gamma radiation is emitted when an atomic nucleus which has too much energy for stability achieves stability by the emission of excess electromagnetic radiation. Some elements, e.g. cobalt 60 are capable of emitting gamma rays of constant energy which have great penetrating qualities and are capable of causing moderately high levels of biological damage at points distant from the source of emission. If it were possible to target a radioactive isotope onto a tumour using a MCA, let us consider the type of radiation that would be best suited for this therapeutic purpose.

The ideal isotope would emit a particle which was capable of causing intense biological damage to any cell it entered. Its range would be limited so that the only cells likely to be affected would be those immediately adjacent to the antibody. This would damage malignant tissue while sparing as much normal tissue as possible. In addition the biological half-life, i.e. the length of time during which the radiation stays in the patient's body, should be relatively short, so the patient is not a radiation hazard to himself or others. Finally, the daughter product of any radioactive decay should itself be inert and harmless as it may stay in the patient's body for many years. Using these criteria an alpha-emitter would seem to be the best isotope type. Recently several isotopes have been made by neutron bombardment of matter in a cyclotron. One cyclotron-produced alpha-emitter is astatine whose half-life is 13 hr. Although production facilities for such an isotope are limited, initial work suggests that this isotope may be successfully conjugated with tumour-directed antibodies. These conjugates can destroy cells with which they come into contact. Once again the importance of the biological properties of the antibody can be seen; any crossreaction with vital normal tissue could cause destruction of essential structures with a catastrophic consequence for the patient. The properties of the antibody and its conjugate after its administration, must be evaluated before widespread clinical application can be contemplated.

Passive radioactive administration

An ingenious method of overcoming some of the theoretical problems with administered radiation has been described. The antibody is conjugated not to a radioactive isotope but to a stable and inert boron atom and is injected into the patient. Assuming again the antibody recognizes and binds to the desired tissue or tumour, with great affinity, it is then possible to bombard the patient or part of the patient with slow or thermal neutrons. The energy of these neutrons is too low to have any significant biological effect on the normal tissue, through which they may pass, but when they encounter the boron atoms the neutrons excite the boron to become an alpha-emitter. This causes great damage in the areas immediately surrounding those tissues containing boron atoms. Unfortunately, slow neutrons have such a low energy that their penetration into the body is limited and thus the application of this technique may be confined to tumours which are relatively superficial. The great advantage of this technique is that it is not necessary to identify each individual deposit of tumour (particularly important in the case of micro metastases). These would be effectively destroyed by the radiation, as long as an antibody was present when neutrons were directed over that area.

Toxins

Some of the most poisonous substances known are produced by plants and bacteria. These toxins occur naturally and are involved in defending the integrity of an organism. It is by toxin production that plants are protected from encroaching parasites that would otherwise find their cell sap a delightful growth medium. Toxins are remarkably potent — several microgrammes being adequate to kill a human, if administered subcutaneously. Some are responsible for the symptoms of disease — tetanus toxin, diphtheria toxin and botulinum toxin. These are produced by bacteria which themselves cause relatively minor local problems but kill by the release of the toxin. Perhaps the most infamous is ricin. In 1978, an alleged Bulgarian spy — Georgyi Markoff — was stabbed with an umbrella at a London bus stop and died mysteriously 2 days later. A tiny pellet containing ricin had been injected into his thigh by an umbrella tip. Certain plant toxins including ricin have a subunit structure that makes them especially suitable for antibody coupling (Fig. 9.2).

Ricin and its related proteins consist of two subunits; an A or active chain and a B or binding chain. For the toxin to kill a mammalian cell, the B chain binds avidly to a galactose containing glycoprotein on the cell surface and the A chain enters the cell. The latter binds to the ribosomes along the endoplasmic reticulum and immediately blocks protein synthesis. The A and B chains are held together by a disulphide linkage coupled through cystine. The two chains can be

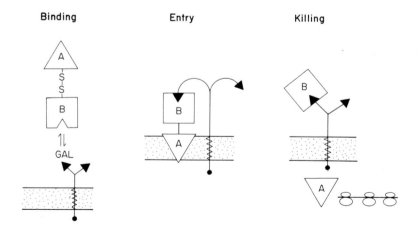

Fig. 9.2. The action of the plant toxin ricin. The B or binding chain binds to the cell surface via a galactose-containing receptor glycoprotein. Once bound the A or active chain is inserted through the membrane. Cell death occurs due to the inhibition of protein synthesis by the A chain.

chemically separated. The isolated A chain has no biological activity as it cannot bind to the cell surface. Similarly, if the B chain is modified in such a way that it can no longer bind — by changing the galactose binding site — then potency is lost. If we take isolated A subunits or whole ricin molecules whose B chain has been suitably damaged, and couple these to a monoclonal antibody of suitable specificity, then at least in theory an ideal conjugate will result. The antibody provides the specificity whilst the ricin acts as a potent warhead — the ultimate in magic bullets.

Of course there are the inevitable snags. There are many chemical problems in stably linking an antibody with a toxin and not abrogating the activity of both molecules. Even after a suitable conjugate has been made, exposure to enzymes in blood and tissue may well cleave the two components apart. Finally the specificity of the antibody in delivering toxin to tumour and not vital normal tissues must be absolute if disastrous clinical effects are to be avoided. Although it is easy to use conjugates to kill tumour cells in culture, it has been a much more difficult exercise in a laboratory animal — and so far unsuccessful in patients. Many experiments are now being performed in this exciting area.

Further reading

Miller R.A., Maloney D.G., McKillop S. & Levy R. (1981) In vivo effects of murine hybridoma monoclonal antibody in a patient with T-cell leukaemia. *Blood*, **58**, 78–86.

Miller R.A., Maloney D.G., Warnke R. & Levy R. (1982) Treatment of B-cell lymphoma with monoclonal anti-idiotype antibody. *New Eng. J. Med..* **306**, 517–522.

Ritz J., Pesando J.M., Sallan S.E., Clavell L.A., Notis-McConarty J., Rosenthal P. & Schlossman S.F. (1981) Serotherapy of acute lymphoblastic leukemia with monoclonal antibody. *Blood*, **58**, 361–372.

Sears H.F., Atkinson B., Mattis J., Ernst C., Herlyn D., Steplewski Z., Hayry P. & Koprowski H. (1982) Phase-I clinical trial of monoclonal antibody in treatment of gastrointestinal tumours. *Lancet*, **i**, 762–765.

Sikora K. & Smedley H.M. (1982) Clinical potential of monoclonal antibodies *Cancer Surveys*, **1**, 521–541.

Sobol R.E., Dillman R.O., Smith J.D., Imai K., Ferrone S., Shawler D., Glassy M.C. & Royston I. (1982) Phase I evaluation of immune monoclonal anti-melanoma antibody in man. In: *Hybridoma in Cancer Diagnosis and Treatment* (Eds M.S. Mitchell & H.F. Oeltgen). Raven Press, New York.

Thorpe P.E. & Ross W.C.J. (1982) The preparation and cytotoxic properties of antibody-toxin conjugate. *Immunol. Rev.* **62**, 1119–1158.

Chapter 10

Human Monoclonal Antibodies*

So far we have considered the production and use of antibodies that have been made by immunizing mice or rats. Such antibodies are already of great use, both to the scientist and the clinician. However, there are problems associated with these antibodies. For several reasons the construction of human antibodies may be advantageous (Table 10.1).

In trying to define tumour-associated antigens a recurring problem has been the relatively low specificity of the resultant monoclonal antibodies. Many of the antigens recognized are present in small quantities on stem cells of normal adult tissues. The immunization of other animals with human tumour material in the preparation of these antibodies, emphasizes certain cell surface components that delineate the 'foreignness' of the animal species rather than the differences between tumour and normal cell. In this way antibodies to blood group substances and histocompatibility antigens arise frequently. If we could immortalize the human immune response to defined antigens then maybe we would have more specific tools for use, both in the laboratory and the clinic. Another problem with specificity arises with interspecies immunization. Although antibodies to certain components result, they do not show the required fine specificity to the different molecular polymorphisms found in certain structures. For example, although many mice have been immunized with proteins of the major human histocompatibility antigens (HLA), few antibodies have been found that recognize fine

Table 10.1. Advantages of human MCA's

1	Possible greater specificity.
2	Allow the dissection of individual components of the human immune system
3	No sensitization on administration to patients for diagnosis or therapy.

*The work described in this chapter was carried out with Dr Thomas Alderson, Mr Jack Phillips and Dr James Watson.

molecular detail adequately enough to distinguish between one HLA type and another. Human monoclonal antibodies should overcome this problem.

As well as improving specificity, the ability to consistently produce human monoclonal antibodies would allow us to study the complex network of the human immune system. We know that in several diseases a disorder of the immune system is likely to be a primary factor. These include debilitating problems such as rheumatoid arthritis, systemic lupus erythematosus, and the whole group of diseases that make up the autoimmune disorders. In many of these conditions abnormal antibodies can be detected in the patient's sera but their relationship to the disease and the aetiological factors in triggering the disease are poorly understood. If we could immortalize the individual components of the network of the immune system, in patients with these diseases, we may be able to shed light on their true cause and this could lead to better treatment methods. In cancer patients we know that an immune response is often elicited by the tumour, but that this immune response is ineffective in destroying the cancer. If we could find out the main factors involved in triggering the immune system, we might be able to do something specifically to stimulate it and so improve the natural defence of a patient against cancer. Similarly in infectious diseases, by increasing our understanding of how the immune system is reacting to a foreign organism, we may be able to curtail the disasterous combination of the death of cells caused by the pathogen, together with an abnormal immune response culminating in the symptoms, signs and pathology that constitute the disease.

A further problem with the conventional rat and mouse monoclonal antibodies when used for either tumour localization or for therapy in cancer or infectious disease, is that their administration to patients may be fraught with danger. They may trigger abnormal immune responses to foreign protein which may result in a sudden fall of blood pressure, and the development of a shock-like state called anaphylaxis. This can be a lethal condition. After repeated administration of foreign animal protein, immune complexes can form which result in kidney damage and joint swelling; the classical features of serum sickness. This was originally seen in the era when passive immunization with foreign animal sera was fashionable in the treatment of infectious diseases. It is caused by the precipitation of the immune complexes in kidneys and joints which results in the activation of macrophages and other destructive cells. Administered human monoclonal antibody would not form complexes and so these destructive effects could not occur. A further advantage of a human antibody is that it may not be neutralized by the formation of host antibodies by recognizing a foreign protein. In theory the administration of large quantities of a single monoclonal human antibody could result in an immune reponse to it. Each antibody differs from the others in its variable or binding site region (idiotype). If enough was administered to a patient, it is possible that an anti-idiotype antibody could be produced. This might disturb the immune network of the patient and cause abrogation of the human monoclonal antibody's effect. This concept is probably only of theoretical interest as no evidence of anti-idiotype antibody formation has been observed, so far, in the few patients that have received human monoclonal antibodies.

Human hybridoma systems

The short history of human monoclonal antibody production has been fraught with technical difficulties. Several novel systems hold out promise. Initial attempts to produce human monoclonal antibodies used the standard mouse and rat myeloma lines for fusion. Human lymphocytes from peripheral blood, lymph nodes, spleen and from within tumours were removed from patients and fused to produce human–mouse or human–rat heterokaryons. These interspecies hybridomas unfortunately lose human chromosomes, eventually ejecting the chromosomes carrying the genes for immunoglobulin production. These genes are present on three different chromosomes; the kappa light chains on chromosome 2; the heavy chains (μ, γ, δ, ϵ and α) on 14; and the lambda light chains on 22. The deletion of human chromosome 14 or the relevant light chain chromosome, will result in cessation of human antibody production and the end of the experiment. After ejection of these chromosomes the ability to produce monoclonal antibodies is lost and therefore a hybrid becomes useless. Early and repetitive cloning of the hybrids can reduce the shedding of human chromosomes, but effort has been placed more recently on the development of stable human/human hybridomas utilizing human myelomas for the fusion process.

Unfortunately, most human myelomas are difficult to grow in

113

tissue culture, having very slow growth rates. Myeloma cells removed from the blood or bone marrow of patients do not grow well in tissue culture. All human tumours are more difficult to grow in tissue culture compared with their animal counterparts. The reason for this is not understood. Despite these difficulties certain myelomas have been adapted to grow in culture at a reasonable rate. Many of these lines, however, are not true myelomas but are lymphoblastoid cells. This means that they are transformed by the Epstein–Barr Virus (EBV), and contain the Epstein–Barr genes within the DNA of the cells. This herpes virus is associated with three human diseases: Burkitt's lymphoma, nasopharyngeal carcinoma and glandular fever (cf. Chapter 5). Lymphoblastoid lines emerge from normal lymphocytes under certain conditions. Their instability is caused by the insertion of EBV oncogenes at appropriate points in their genome. EBV-transformed cells tend to grow very slowly in tissue culture and produce only small amounts of immunoglobulin. Some, however, have adapted well to tissue culture, and have also been made azaguanine resistant. This allows the self-destruct mechanism to operate when the hybridized cells are placed in HAT-selective medium.

There have been difficulties in human hybridization with some of the myelomas that investigators have produced over the last few years. One problem has been infection with a mycoplasma, a microorganism that causes considerable havoc in tissue culture laboratories. The available cell lines are listed in Table 10.2. The ideal properties of a human fusion system include a high frequency of fusion; a high cloning efficiency; the ability to grow rapidly in nonstringent serum conditions; and no secretion of myeloma or lymphoid

Table 10.2. Human monoclonal antibody production

Lymphocyte source	Myeloma	Target antigen
PBL	TEPC-15	—
CLL	NS1	—
Spleen	NS1	Influenza virus
PBL	GM1500	Measles virus
Nodes	NS1	Breast carcinoma
Nodes	NS1	Lung carcinoma
Spleen	U266	DNCB
Tumour	HMy2	Glioma

cell immunoglobulin and yet maintain the production of large amounts of immunoglobulin after fusion to suitable lymphocyte donors. The continued production by hybrids of immunoglobulins, coded for by the parent myeloma poses problems, both in their detection and in the strength of the resulting antibodies. Heavy and light immunoglobulin chains produced within a single cell will mix randomly. If these chains are coded for by both myeloma and lymphocyte gene sequences, mixed molecules will occur. It can be calculated that for a standard IgG-secreting hybrid, only one in eight complete immunoglobulin molecules will be a replica of the lymphocyte-coded IgG of interest (Fig. 10.1). One of the best lines available so far is the

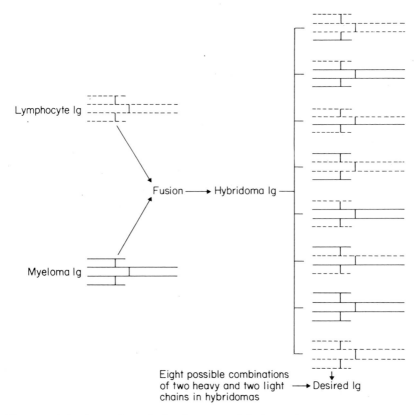

Fig. 10.1. The formation of mixed immunoglobulin molecules by the mixing of heavy and light chains coded by myeloma and lymphocyte genes in the hybridoma. This reduces the affinity of the supernatant to any antigen.

115

LICR/LON/HMy2; a derivative of the ARH77 human myeloma, that was cultured in the U.S.A. in 1975. This line expresses EBV surface antigens and therefore must be catagorized as a lymphoblastoid line rather than a true myeloma. Reasonable fusion frequencies have been obtained, but unfortunately the immunoglobulin secretion rate is low. There are several other lines available which all have their own individual problems. The search is on in many laboratories for more ideal fusion systems.

EBV transformation

Another method of immortalizing and cloning lymphocytes, in such a way that human monoclonal antibodies are produced, is to infect lymphocytes deliberately with EB virus. In this way lymphoblastoid lines can be grown from lymphocytes which hopefully are producing the antibody of interest. This is not as easy as it seems. One of the main problems is the slow growth rate of EB-transformed cells and the difficulty in growing them up from single cells during the cloning process. However, several groups have now made human monoclonal antibodies using EBV transformation. Antibodies against tetanus toxoid, influenza virus and the rhesus blood group antigens on human red blood cells are currently available. One approach is to initially transform cells with EBV; select those with the required antibody specificity, prior to formal cloning and subsequently immortalize by cell fusion using a hybridoma system. In this way the cloning step comes in the last part of the process. Screening assays are performed earlier to make it highly probable that clones of interest will emerge. The production of human monoclonal antibodies against human tetanus toxoid in this way is used as an example.

All fusion techniques require a selection process to curtail the growth of unfixed cells, in this case lymphoblastoid lines. After checking that these lines are indeed producing anti-tetanus antibodies, a hybridization to a myeloma can be performed. Some selection process must now be devised to prevent the continued growth of the lymphoblastoid line after fusion. HAT sensitivity is of no use in this situation, for fusions with a HAT-sensitive myeloma will result in the death of all cells when placed in HAT. Unless the HPRT gene exists in at least one of the fusion partners, then no hybrid can grow.

Another selective marker, ouabain resistance, can be introduced into lymphoblastoid cells by growing them in increasing concentrations of this drug. Ouabain is a cardiac glycoside which stimulates the contractility of heart muscle. This drug inhibits the membrane sodium-potassium ATPase in normal cells. This surface enzyme is responsible for maintaining the electrolyte state of the cell. Ouabain-resistant, EB-transformed, antibody-producing cells are fused to a HAT-sensitive myeloma system. Subsequently the hybrids are grown up in both HAT and ouabain. Lymphocytes are obtained from suitably immunized individuals. Tetanus toxoid is administered intramuscularly on several occasions over a 3-month period. Enrichment for the peripheral blood lymphocytes, involved in anti-tetanus antibody production, can be achieved by pulling out those cells bearing the antibody on their cell surface. This can be performed most precisely by using fluorescein-coupled toxin and a cell sorter. Cells are mixed with the fluorescein coupled toxin for 1 hr at 4°C and then repeatedly washed. Those cells bearing the antibody on the surface will bind the toxin and so will fluoresce in ultraviolet light after washing. The cells are passed in tiny single droplets through the nozzle of a flow cytometer. A ultraviolet light source excites each droplet and the emitted fluorescence is recorded by a detector at right angles to the source. An ingenious electrostatic deflector system coupled to a computer, enables the droplets containing the cells that fluoresce to be deviated into one test tube whilst the remaining non-fluorescent cells are not deflected. In this way the antigen-recognizing cells can be concentrated. EB virus can be obtained from supernatants from EBV-secreting cell lines and used to infect the selected cells. After infection and fusion, the screening and cloning procedures are identical to those previously described. The combination of EBV transformation with hybridization is likely to yield hybrids that retain the advantages of both systems.

Human monoclonal antibodies to cancer

The production of human monoclonal antibodies to cancer cells has elicited great interest because of the difficulty in producing tumour-specific antibodies in animals. Several groups have now described human antibody activity against a variety of tumour types. Lymphocytes are taken from patients at a time when they are likely to be producing antibodies to their own tumour. An example are the lymphocytes in lymph nodes draining the site of the tumour, such as axillary nodes in breast cancer, or thoracic nodes in lung cancer. Another method is to take lymphocytes from within a tumour, to separate these from the tumour cells and use them for fusion. Lymphocytes in large numbers áre not normally present in tissue and thus their presence in a tumour suggests that they are playing some role in host defence against the cancer. Human monoclonal antibodies have been produced for a variety of tumour types. To illustrate some of the techniques and problems involved our own experience is detailed below.

We collected tumour material and, where available, regional lymph nodes from patients undergoing surgery for a variety of cancers. One gram of tumour was cut into 1-ml cubes using fine scissors in tissue culture medium and frozen in liquid nitrogen. Pieces of corresponding normal tissue, where available, were similarly stored. Lymphocytes were purified from peripheral blood using standard techniques. Lymph nodes were teased apart by forceps and dead cells removed. Intratumoural lymphocytes were collected in a similar manner.

We chose to use the LICR/LON/HMy2 line for fusion. This is a human lymphoblastoid line which grows rapidly in normal tissue culture medium and dies in HAT. This line was adapted for growth on serum-free medium and cloned. Several clones were tested for their ability to fuse with peripheral blood lymphocytes and one chosen for further study. For each fusion, the recovered lymphocytes and a constant number of 10^7 myeloma cells were suspended in serum-free medium, mixed, and centrifuged in a conical-bottomed plastic centrifuge tube. The supernatant was drained off completely. Polyethylene glycol (PEG) and dimethyl sulphoxide (DMSO) in serum-free medium was added to the pellet, and the cells were gently resuspended using the tip of the pipette. After 1 min, PEG without DMSO was added and the mixture stirred gently. Medium containing fetal calf serum (FCS) was added dropwise, and the mixture rocked for a further 4 min. More medium with 10% FCS was slowly added, and the mixture was taken up carefully in a wide bore pipette, and dispensed equally into each of ninety-six wells in plates. One millilitre of medium with 10% FCS was added to each well. After 24 hr the medium was replaced by selective medium containing HAT, with 20% FCS. The selective medium was renewed daily for the first 2 weeks. Hybrid clones visibly appeared in the wells between 3 to 6 weeks after fusion. Supernatants from well-grown wells were taken for testing and stored at 4°C. Following dilution cloning, immunoglobulin secreted by the hybridomas was assayed by a sensitive radioimmunoassay using Ig-chain-specific antibodies. Bulk supernatants from cloned hybrids were grown in roller bottles in Iscove's serum-free medium supplemented with insulin. Bulk supernatants were harvested and concentrated using an ultrafiltration unit.

The detection of low concentrations of specific human immunoglobulins is an essential prerequisite for the development of human hybridoma systems. The assays currently available for human immunoglobulins include radial immunodiffusion, electroimmunoassay, antibody-coupled red cell lysis, and double antibody inhibition radioimmunoassay. These assays are not all sensitive in the microgram range and often show loss of specificity when the concentration of immunoglobulin is low. A rapid solid-phase radioimmunoassay which is chain specific at concentrations of immunoglobulin below 20 ng/ml was developed. Commercially available polyclonal and monoclonal antibodies were used in this, thus making the assay readily available for any laboratory. Rabbit anti-human immunoglobulin antiserum was obtained by immunizing rabbits with purified human immunoglobulins. The antiserum was diluted in phosphate-buffered saline (PBS) and aliquots added to round-bottomed, ninety-six-well vinyl plastic plates and incubated overnight at 4°C. These plates were subsequently washed in medium four times by flicking the contents of the wells into a sink and replacing with medium. The wells were incubated for 1 hr with medium containing albumen. This ensured complete saturation of the plastic binding sites by albumen in the complete medium. The sensitivity of the technique was determined by titrating human serum containing known amounts of different immunoglobulins starting at 50 μg/ml in 50 μl. After incubating for 1 hr at room temperature the plates were washed in the manner previously described. Fifty microlitres of chain-specific monoclonal mouse anti-human immunoglobulin was added, prepared by immunizing mice with three injections of the relevant immunoglobulin and subsequent fusion of the mouse spleen lymphocytes. After cloning, the line was grown as an ascites tumour. Monoclonal antibodies were used at a concentration of 1/50000 (approximately 1 ng/ml of mouse immunoglobulin). After 1 hr of

119

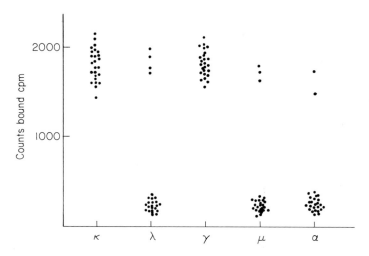

Fig. 10.2. Radioimmunoassay for different Ig chains in thirty-five supernatants from a human fusion. Counts above 200 cpm indicate presence of Ig chain.

incubation with the relevant monoclonal antibodies, the plates were washed and rat anti-mouse immunoglobulin coupled to [125] I was added. After a final incubation and washing in complete medium, the plates were air dried, the wells cut with a hot wire, and counted in a gamma counter. This technique is very similar to that described in Chapter 2 for screening mouse or rat monoclonal antibodies. The secretion of new immunoglobulin types by the hybrids could be detected easily (Fig. 10.2).

The DNA content of the hybrids was determined using a flow cytometer. This remarkable instrument allows the precise quantitation of DNA within a single cell as it passes through a flow nozzle (cf. Chapter 6). The cells are stained with ethidium bromide, a dye which intercalates between the bases of the DNA of each cell. The more DNA present, the more ethidium bromide will intercalate. Cells are diluted and passed in droplets of fluid through a jet. The amount of fluorescence emitted by each cell is picked up by a detector. The more ethidium bromide present, the more light emitted. Figure 10.3 shows the measurement of the DNA content by a flow cytometer in hybrids from lymphocytes taken from a patient with a malignant brain tumour.

A large number of hybrids were manufactured and their super-

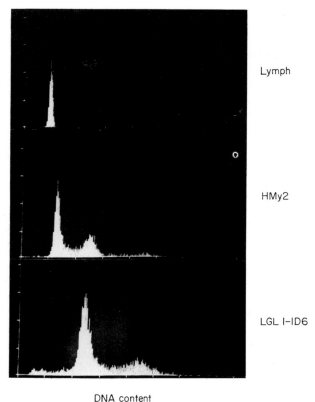

Lymph

HMy2

LGL I–ID6

DNA content

Fig. 10.3. DNA content by flow cytometry of lymphocytes; HMy2 myeloma cells and a human-human hybridoma (LGL1-1D6) showing increased content of hybridoma.

natants collected. Antibodies were initially screened for binding activity against the cell line most appropriate to the source of donor lymphocyte. An example of the assay used in such a screen is shown in Figure 10.4. Despite the sensitivity of the binding assay, the counts bound are low. After concentration, however, titration curves were obtained. These curves show clear binding of antibody. The specificity of binding was determined using a panel of tumour cell lines. Peripheral blood lymphocytes and red blood cells from normal donors were used as controls. All the antibodies isolated so far bind to a variety of cell types and are not individually tumour-specific.

121

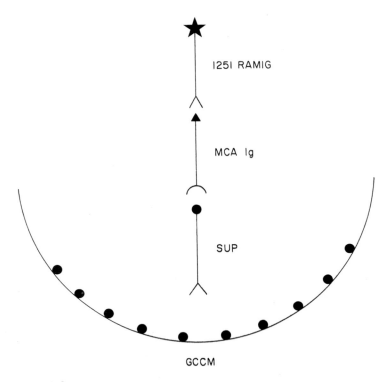

Fig. 10.4. Schematic of binding assay for detecting human anti-tumour MCA's. GCCM is a glioma cell line.

We have demonstrated that lymphocytes from patients with several tumour types can be successfully fused with a human myeloma line to produce stable hybridomas. These hybridomas secrete immunoglobulins, several of which have been found to show binding to tumour cell lines in an indirect radioimmunoassay. Evidence for hybridization, rather than by outgrowth of lymphoblastoid lines from the patients lymphocytes, is provided by the continued secretion of HMy2 immunoglobulin as well as the new lymphocyte immunoglobulin in cloned hybridomas. Flow cytometric DNA analysis shows the stably increased DNA content, characteristic of hybrids (cf. Fig. 10.3). Formal karyotypic analysis has been performed on hybridomas derived from HMy2 which confirms a stably increased chromosome number.

There are several problems with the hybridoma system. Firstly, the low fusion frequency results in a large workload to produce small numbers of hybrids. Several methods have been used in attempts to increase this frequency. These have included provision of feeder cells and secondary *in vitro* stimulation by either antigen (tumour cells) or by pokeweed mitogen. No increase in fusion frequency was observed. A second problem is the continued secretion of the HMy2 κ- and γ-immunoglobulin chains by the hybridomas. A true assessment of the numbers of hybrids secreting Ig coded for by genes of the donor lymphocytes is thus difficult. Furthermore, mixed antibody molecules comprised of chains coded by both myeloma or lymphocyte genes will occur. Such molecules will have reduced antibody activity. A third problem is the low antibody secretion rate of between 1 and 10 μg/ml. Large amounts of tissue culture supernatant must be concentrated in order to increase the signal-to-noise ratio in the radioimmunoassay. The poorly developed endoplasmic reticulum, in all hybrids examined by electron microscopy, suggests that the rate of protein synthesis may well be limiting. The initial screen for anti-tumour antibody activity may be unable to detect small amounts of weak antibodies (cf. Fig. 10.4). Finally, the low anti-tumour binding activity hinders the analysis of specificity of the resulting antibodies. The specificity studies on twelve antibodies shows a wide range of binding to different tumour cell lines. It is of interest that none of the antibodies bound to the benign fibroblast line (MRC5), normal red cells, or peripheral blood lymphocytes.

Use in tumour localization

Two of these antibodies, one against lung cancer and one against glioma, were labelled with a radioactive isotope, ^{131}I, as described in Chapter 8 and used in attempts to localize lung and brain cancer. A 21-year-old girl presenting with a 6-month history of headaches of increasing severity, together with progressive dementia was found to have a large glioma as shown on a CT scan. An operation was performed, the tumour excised and lymphocytes sent to the laboratory. The patient then received post-operative radiotherapy in order to try to prevent tumour recurrence. From this patient we were successful in obtaining several monoclonal antibodies, one of which bound with a reasonable affinity to glioma cells. Unfortunately, 6 months following

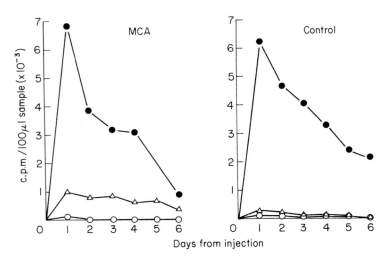

Fig. 10.5. Distribution of ¹³¹I-labelled human anti-glioma (MCA) and control monoclonal IgG (CONTROL) in a 21-year-old patient with a large recurrent glioma. ●, Serum; △, tumour cyst fluid; ○, cerebrospinal fluid.

the primary excision, the patient's presenting symptoms returned. Investigations revealed a recurrent cystic tumour at exactly the same site as the initial disease. A second operation was performed to reduce the pressure that had built up within the cranial cavity causing severe headaches. Two cannulae were inserted to reduce this pressure, one into the cerebro-spinal fluid cavity surrounding the brain and the other within the tumour cyst fluid itself.

One milligram of purified radiolabelled antibody was injected intravenously and samples of blood, CSF and tumour cyst fluid removed daily following this injection. Brain scan images were obtained using a rectilinear scanner which recorded the total counts emitted and the ¹³¹I distribution. Three weeks subsequent to this, a control monoclonal immunoglobulin was given (which did not bind to glioma cells), labelled in exactly the same way to make sure that any uptake in the tumour was not an artifact of tumour blood flow. Figure 10.5 shows the radioactive counts in serum, CSF and tumour cyst fluids following the administration of monoclonal antibody and control immunoglobulins. There was no significant difference between the counts in the serum or CSF after the administration of antibody or control protein. However, within the tumour cyst fluid the label from

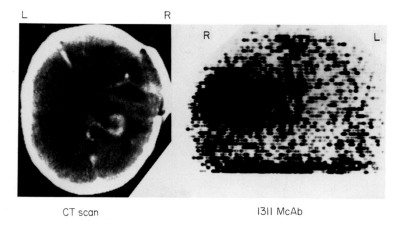

CT scan   I3II McAb

Fig. 10.6. Computerized tomography and rectilinear scans after the administraticn of ^{131}I human MCA to a patient with a malignant glioma. The CT scan, by convention, is represented by looking down from above. The rectilinear scan is a frontal view.

the monoclonal antibody persisted for more than 6 days. The level of activity was five times higher than that of the control protein. These results were borne out by external counting and rectilinear scanning (Fig. 10.6). Similar results have now been obtained in lung cancer where tumour uptake of human monoclonal antibody has been detected by scanning.

Continuous administration

To study the feasibility of continuous administration of human monoclonal antibodies directed against glioma we designed a chamber which enables hybridoma cells to be cultured in the subcutaneous tissue. This chamber allows antibodies to diffuse out, and nutrients and oxygen necessary for continued cell viability to diffuse in. Cells are unable to traverse the membrane pores of the device, so there is no risk that malignant cells put in the chamber can spread (Fig. 10.7). The chamber has now been inserted into patients with recurrent glioma, in whom the kinetics of internally labelled antibody release have been monitored.

The cylindrical diffusion chamber was constructed of a synthetic

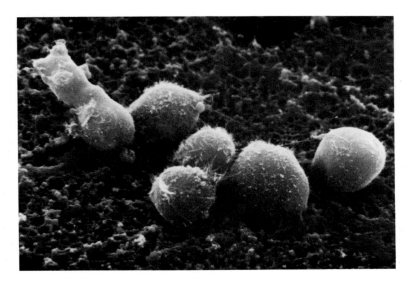

Fig. 10.7. Scanning electron microscopy of human hybridomas growing on the millipore filter of a subcutaneous chamber. The cell on the left is dividing.

homopolymer. The upper section contained an outlet and inlet hole into which were inserted needles. This assembly screws into the lower cylindrical section which has an internal and external flange at the base. The internal flange holds a 'millipore' filter. The external flange enables the chamber to be immobilized in the subcutaneous tissue. The filter allows the free diffusion of large molecules, but not of cells, between the chamber and the patient's extracellular fluid (Plate 4).

10^7 hybridoma cells which were pulse-labelled with 100 μCi of (4,5-3H) lysine monohydrochloride (specific activity 80 μCi/mmol) were also placed in the chamber. Serum samples were collected from the patient at regular intervals after the insertion of the chamber, and ^{3}H counts determined by scintillation counting. Release of tritiated monoclonal antibody from the chamber into the blood stream, occurred in the 3 days after injection of pulse-labelled cells into the chamber. Intact labelled antibody was detected in the tumour cyst fluid. The device remained *in situ* for 3 months and caused no problems — there was no evidence of infection or of an inflammatory response around the chamber and no evidence of spread of hybridoma cells outside the chamber. There was no change in the patient's serum EBV titre. This sort of device can be used to study the long-term effects of this and other monoclonal antibodies.

Conclusion

It is clear that human monoclonal antibodies are feasible, although difficult to obtain. Tremendous efforts are being invested in their production and over the next few years we should see a wide spectrum of different antibodies for use in clinical medicine. Most laboratories at the moment are busy trying to develop better fusion systems before embarking upon large-scale production and screening programmes which obviously consume much time and effort. It can be seen that there are many technical problems in the production of human monoclonal antibodies. It is really too early to know whether all the current efforts will result in biologically interesting molecules with fundamental and clinical potential, or just additional reagents of little difference from the other animal antibodies that can be obtained with significantly less effort.

Further reading

Croce C.M., Linnenbach A., Hall W., Steplewski Z. & Koprowski H. (1980) Production of human hybridomas secreting antibodies to measles virus. *Nature*, **288**, 488.

Kaplan H. & Olsson L. (1980) Human-human hybridomas producing monoclonal antibodies of predefined specificity. *Proc. Natl. Acad. Sci. (USA)*, **77**, 5429.

Kozbur D. & Roder J.C. (1983) The production of monoclonal antibodies from human lymphocytes. *Immunol. Today*, **4**, 72–79.

Sikora K., Alderson T. & Ellis J. (1983) Human hybridomas from patients with maligant disease. *Br. J. Cancer*, **47**, 135–145.

Sikora K., Alderson T., Phillips J. & Watson J.V. (1982) Human hybridomas from malignant gliomas. *Lancet*, **i**, 11–14.

Watson J.V., Alderson T., Phillips J. & Sikora K. (1983) Subcutaneous culture chamber for continuous infusion of monoclonal antibodies. *Lancet*, **i** 99–100.

Glossary

Affinity. The intrinsic binding power of an antibody combining site with a single antigenic determinant.

Allergy. An altered state of immune reactivity usually due to agents in the environment such as animal hair or grass pollens.

Antibody. Immunoglobulin molecules produced by animals in response to exposure to an antigen. Antibodies specifically combine with antigens.

Ascites. Fluid in the peritoneal cavity. Only tiny amounts are normally present. If myeloma or hybridoma cells are present then several mls may gather in a mouse.

Autoradiography. The direct apposition of radioactive material (e.g. labelled antibodies on their target antigens) and a photographic emulsion or film. The distribution of radioactivity can be detected by developing the emulsion or film.

Avidity. The total combining power of an antibody molecule with its antigen. This depends on both the number of binding sites and their affinity.

Bursa of Fabricius. Lymphoid organ which processes B-lymphocytes in birds.

Clone. A family of cells derived by cell division of one single parent. Such cells must be completely identical.

CSF. Cerebrospinal fluid – the fluid bathing the brain and spinal cord.

Determinant. The site of an antigen that is recognised by and binds to an antibody.

Epitope. As determinant.

Feeder Cells. Cells whose function is to maintain the growth (usually by secreting growth factors) of other cells.

Genome. The total complement of genetic material within a cell.

Fusion. The intimate mixing of cells to produce a hybrid cell.

HAT. Medium containing hypoxanthine, aminopterin, and thymidine to stop myeloma cell growth after fusion.

HPRT. Hypoxanthine phosphoribosyl transferase.

Hybridoma. Immortalized fusion product of B-lymphocyte and myeloma cells.

Idiotype. The individual antigenic determinant produced by the antigen binding site on an antibody.

Immunization. Stimulation of the immune system by the administration of an antigen.

Isotopes. Radioactive forms of atoms that can be incorporated into biological molecules such as antibodies.

Karyotype. Chromosomal pattern detected by spreading out chromosomes in cells during mitosis.

Metastasis. A focus of cancer distant from its primary site of origin.

Mitogen. A substance that causes lymphocytes to undergo cell division.

Monoclonal. A single clone.

Mutation. An alteration in the genetic constitution of a cell.

Myeloma. A tumour of immunoglobulin secreting B-lymphocytes.

PEG. Polyethylene glycol.

Plasma cell. Fully differentiated antibody producing B lymphocyte.

Plasmacytoma. As myeloma.

Reticuloendothelial system. A diffuse organ containing phagocytic cells involved in clearance of immune complexes and other particles.

SDS–PAGE. Sodium dodecyl sulphate – poly acrylamide gel electrophoresis.

Spent medium. Medium from growing cells which contains secreted growth factors.

Titre. Reciprocal value of the highest possible dilution of an antibody.

Xenograft. The grafting of tissue to an immunosuppressed animal of a different species: a convenient method to grow human tumours in experimental animals for further study.

Index

INDEX

INDEX